Laughter

Laughter

Eric Smadja

ISBN 978-1-84890-119-3

College Publications
Scientific Director: Dov Gabbay
Managing Director: Jane Spurr

http://www.collegepublications.co.uk

Original cover design by Laraine Welch
Printed by Lightning Source, Milton Keynes, UK

Table of Contents

Chapter IV: **Socio-cultural Facets**

INTRODUCTION

The discourse about laughter that has now become traditional, "popular," seems to summon to mind three principal characteristics of laughter: its specifically human nature; its structural relationship to the joy and pleasure procured by what is laughable, making laughter an indicator of "good health;" its automatic, reflexive aspect combined with its intellectual self-evidence with regard to any potential questioning by the one engaging in it.

"Laughter is properly human," Aristotle said, [1] an idea later picked up by François Rabelais.[2] Having then become a commonplace, this statement established a clear break between the animal realm and human beings, nature and culture. Laughter properly belongs to the human species and to culture without having any observable, identifiable antecedents in the closest relatives of human beings, the anthropoid apes.

Other than that, laughter points to the affect joy and the pleasure procured by what is comical. Its mere manifestation suffices to suggest or hint at this affect and the laughable nature of the stimuli triggering it. "One laughs when one is happy, because one is happy, when a laughable situation brings us pleasure." Laughter seems structurally linked to joy, to pleasure, and is a response to laughable messages. Actually, it suggests good mental health.

Finally, its "impulsive," "convulsive" qualities bring to mind notions of automatism, of reflexive reaction, even mechanical execution void of any prior ideation and mental operation. Laughter is neither verbalized nor meditated. It happens and is engaged in. Automatism and mental self-evidence call to mind a reflection that Lévi-Strauss once made concerning the unconscious nature of collective phenomena. He formulated his ideas in the introduction to his work *Structural Anthropology*:

> There is rarely any doubt that the unconscious reasons for practicing a custom or sharing a belief are remote from the reasons given to justify them. Even in our society, table manners, social etiquette, fashion of dress, and many of our moral, political, and religious attitudes are scrupulously observed by everyone, although their real origin and function are not often critically examined. We act and think according to habit.[3]

---

[1] Aristotle, *On the Parts of Animals* III, 10.

[2] François Rabelais, "Rabelais to the Reader," *Gargantua*.

[3] Claude Lévi-Strauss, "Introduction: History and Anthropology," *Structural Anthropology, Volume 2*, trans. Monique Layton, Chicago: University of Chicago Press, 1983.

Like Lévi-Strauss, we could also consider laughter to be an unconscious social practice experienced as a habit by those engaging in it and a matter of secondary rationalizations or elaborations of ideas.

This traditional discourse conveying popular impressions has gone hand in hand with   the interest that numerous scholars have displayed in the phenomenon of laughter. Indeed, philosophers, psychologists, ethologists, medical doctors, in particular, have expressed ideas, certain ones of which have been structured into explanatory theories claiming general applicability. In fact, this is rather a matter of partial depictions of the same phenomenon, thus producing a body of knowledge useable at a later stage for the purposes of elaborating a synthetic depiction.

These two types of discourse seem unsatisfactory to me. The first one seems to obscure two fundamental aspects of laughter: its historicity and the complexity of its determinism. By atomizing its object, the second one, being merely analytic, offers a reductionist vision having little heuristic value.

Like Marcel Mauss, in his essay on the techniques of the body, I think that all human behavior, facial mimicry or other "bodily techniques" must be the object of a multidisciplinary approach involving biological, psychological and socio-cultural considerations . Indeed, positioned at the highest level of the evolution of the animal realm, human beings have incorporated the different stages and attainments of phylogenesis while breaking with, and clearly distancing themselves from, their closest relations the anthropoid apes by making "two major innovations," by the emergence of a twofold life, mental and cultural, encoded by a well-developed system of linguistic signs. However, the human phylogenetic legacy transmitted by the genome has been preserved and assimilated into new specifically human attainments (a complex psyche and culture) in order to participate in behavioral schemes that are unique in terms of the complexity of their determinism, their functional multi-purposefulness and their multiple meanings. It thus becomes urgent to think in terms of the "total person"

Let us cite Mauss'words in this regard:

> And I concluded that it was not possible to have a clear idea of all these facts about running, swimming, etc., unless one introduced a triple consideration instead of a single consideration, be it mechanical and physical like an anatomical and physiological theory of walking or on the contrary psychological or sociological. It is the triple viewpoint, that of the total man, that is needed.[1]

---

[1] Marcel Mauss, "Techniques of the Body," *Techniques, Technology and Civilisation*, Nathan Schlanger (ed.), New York: Durkheim Press, 2006.

So, I believe that making laughter more intelligible requires turning to the conceptual set of tools and the unique methods of the following disciplines: ethology, medicine, cognitive psychology, psychoanalysis and anthropology. One of the modes of their interaction may be supplied by the idea of communication.

Indeed, traditionally perceived as being a facial emotional expression, laughter is fundamentally a mode of nonverbal communication of different types of affective messages among which figure, in the first place, joy and pleasure, but also aggressiveness and anxiety.

In fact, this idea of communication could well be the unifying concept by means of which laughter's biological, psychological, pathological and socio-cultural facets may be envisaged.

In Chapter I, I provide three classic definitions of laughter. I cite a certain number of uses of the word 'laughter' as found in various different expressions of the English language and then I engage in a philosophical exploration of the ideas of thinkers from Antiquity up until Henri Bergson.

Philosophers are in fact pertinent inquirers in search of answers, and laughter as Ludovic Dugas wrote,[1] has been the object of numerous reflections, certain ones of which have been structured into theories. They thus elucidate the complexity of laughter.

In Chapter II, ethology tackles the phenomenology of laughter and strives to recount its ontogenesis as well as its phylogenesis, factors of its historicity.

The aim of Chapter III is to look at the external and internal factors contributing to triggering and producing laughter. The external determinism would correspond to the laughable (which is also intra-psychic), while the complex, multiple, internal determinants include the processes of psychic and cerebral production, as well as those of motor and phonatory realization. Investigating them requires recourse to data supplied by neurology, psychiatry and psychoanalysis.

By the end of the second and third chapters, the biological and psychic encoding of laughter will have been outlined.

Finally, Chapter IV studies the different modes of a socio-cultural approach to laughter once reinserted into its "natural" milieu, which is the social

---

[1] Ludovic Dugas, *Psychologie du Rire (1902)*, Whitefish MT: Kessinger Publishing, 2010.

and cultural life of a historically determined group. The parameters of its cultural encoding will be defined. I shall use ethnographic facts to set out my own view of the relationships between laughter and the laughable forming a laughable-laughter system of communication. Laughter will then occupy an intermediary position between the laughable system of communication and that of individual and social emotional expressions.

I hope that by the end of this exploratory voyage through the arcana of laughter, the pertinence of the multidisciplinary light I will have shed on the subject may be such as to generate cogent discourse finally offering a synthetic, therefore new, view having definite heuristic value.

Since 1993, the year of the first French edition of this work, interest in laughter has grown considerably. The mass media and public opinion have developed and conveyed their own views accompanied by rather peremptory and prescriptive talk of the kind: "We live in a society and in times in which we do not laugh much. Laughter is good for one and therapeutic. We have to laugh more." So laughter associations, clubs and schools have been created and proliferated widely. Although this contemporary socio-cultural phenomenon is a particularly interesting one, it will not be explored here. Now, let us "make way for laughter."

LITERARY FACETS AND PHILOSOPHICAL SPECULATIONS

I.   Definitions

Consulting three major English language dictionaries, we read:

Laugh v. (*Oxford English Dictionary*) "To make the sounds and movements of the face usual in expressing joy, mirth, amusement, or and (sometimes) derision; to have the same reaction in response to being tickled; to emit laughter. Also in extended use: to feel joy, mirth, amusement, or derisions without such accompanying sounds and movements."

Laugh v. (*Webster's Dictionary*) "To make a convulsive or chuckling noise excited by merriment or pleasure."

Laugh v. (*Random House Dictionary*) "To express emotion, as mirth, pleasure, derision, or nervousness, with an audible, vocal expulsion of air from the lungs that can range from a loud burst of sound to a series of quiet chuckles."

So, in these dictionary definitions laughter appears as a facial expression expressing a feeling of gaiety and having two facets, visual and auditory.

II.   Uses of the verb "to laugh" in the English language

In the English language we encounter numerous expressions using the verb "to laugh" that, displaying a diversity of meanings, contrast with the one-dimensionality of the behavioral response. Let us take a look at this multiplicity of uses of the verb as they appear in quotes from the works of famous writers cited in that definitive record of the English language, the *Oxford English Dictionary*.[1]

- To laugh until one cries. Joseph Conrad, *Lord Jim* xiii. 139, "He made us laugh till we cried, and would tiptoe amongst us and say, 'It's all very well for you beggars to laugh.'"

- Not to know whether to laugh or cry. Charles Dickens, *Martin Chuzzlewit* (1844) xii. 150, "It was a toss-up with Tom Pinch whether he should laugh or cry."

---

[1] "laugh, v.," Oxford English Dictionary, Third edition, June 2011, online version September 2011. http://www.oed.com/view/Entry/106250, accessed 25 October 2011.

- To laugh one's head off. Mark Twain, *Burlesque Autobiography*. 6, "He could imitate anybody's hand so closely that it was enough to make a person laugh his head off to see it."

- To laugh oneself sick. H. C. Witwer, *Leather Pushers* xii. 325, "I'll wager she's laughing herself sick right now."

- Laugh! I thought I'd die. Fannie Hurst, *Anatomy of Me, A Wonderer in Search of Herself*, I. 15, "I could listen to Mrs. Hurst talk all day! Laugh! I thought I'd die! The way she says things."

- To laugh upon: to regard with affection or goodwill, to smile at or upon. Samuel Pepys, *Diary* 7 Jan. (1976) IX. 410, "A bold merry slut, who lay laughing there upon the people."

- Don't make me laugh. J. B. Priestley, *It's Old Country* xiii, 142, "I'll never believe there was anything between him and Mum—' 'Don't make me laugh,' Vic said giving Tom a wink."

- To laugh at, to mock, deride, to make fun of. Charlotte Brontë, *Professor*, "'I wonder whether you'll be still out of place!' he laughed, as mockingly, as heartlessly as Mephistopheles."

- To laugh down. Edward Chodorov, *Kind Lady* II. 58, "I laughed her down of course–told her she was a silly woman, I insulted her frightfully."

- To laugh at oneself first. Robert L'Estrange, translator *Of Anger* viii. 83 in *Seneca's Morals Abstracted* (1679), "No Man was ever ridiculous to others, that laught at himself first."

- To laugh in a person's face: to show open contempt for a person, esp. with scornful mockery or laughter; to deride, ridicule, or scoff at a person blatantly. Thackeray, *Vanity Fair* ii. 13, "Rebecca laughed in her face, with a horrid sarcastic demoniacal laughter, that almost sent the schoolmistress into fits."

- To laugh in the face of: to show open contempt for something, especially a known hazard or encumbrance. Samuel Taylor Coleridge, *Lett.* (1895) 209, "Laugh in the faces of gloom and ill-lookingness."

- To laugh away, Lord Byron, *Marino Faliero* VI. i. 10, "I strove To laugh the thought away."

- To laugh up one's sleeve: to laugh to oneself, to nurse inward feelings of amusement or derision. Matthew Arnold, *Empedocles on Etna* I.ii, "The Gods laugh in their sleeve To watch man doubt and fear."

- To laugh on the other side of one's mouth: to laugh bitterly or ruefully, to suffer reverse of circumstances after feeling satisfaction or confidence about something. B. H. Malkin, translation of Alain-René Le Sage, *Adventures of Gil Blas* I. II. V. 227, "We were made to laugh on the other side of our mouths by an unforeseen occurrence."

- He laughs best who laughs last: "Your Grace knows the French proverb, 'He laughs best who laughs last.'" Sir Walter Scott, *Peveril* IV. iii. 49.

- Of an inanimate object: to appear lively with movement, sound, or the play of light and color, as if expressing joyous feeling: Alexander Pope's translation of Homer's *Odyssey* I. III. 601, "In the dazzling goblet laughs the wine."

So it is that laughter can be multi-faceted. It can display benevolence, arrogance, hostility, derision, but it above all seems to express a certain ambivalence.

III. Philosophical speculations

Many philosophers and literary figures have formulated their reflections on laughter and the laughable. Some of them have developed and structured them and so elaborated theories.

We shall therefore explore what they have said. Then at the end of this speculative itinerary, I shall present the great conceptualizations of laughter that have become classic.

However, it is important to point out that all these pronouncements from different thinkers and times are, above all, not only to be reinserted back into their historically determined socio-cultural framework, generative of a quite unique system of ideas and values, but are also to be integrated into the conceptual system constructed by each one of the inquirers concerned.

I am indeed aware of, and lucid about, the dangers involved in uprooting their speculations on laughter and the laughable.

1. **Thinkers of Antiquity**

A) *Two Greek thinkers: Plato and Aristotle*

a) Plato. It is essentially in the passage of the *Philebus* concerning mixed pleasures that, through Socrates' dialogue with Protarchus, Plato presents his conceptions of laughter and the laughable.[1]

Above all, laughing is a pleasure. But this pleasure can be mixed with pain in a variety of circumstances, among them ridicule and mockery.

Envy[2] is "painful for the soul," and the envious person, according to Plato, obviously rejoices in the misfortunes of others. Thus the laughter associated with ridiculousness, with mockery would be based on envy.[3]

But what is involved in ridicule and what is the ill fortune of others about which one can rejoice?

Ridiculousness is an evil consisting in ignorance, in false opinion and, therefore, in the illusion that weak, harmless subjects display with respect to themselves in the three areas of wealth, the body and the mind. They see themselves as rich, handsome and wise, and we see them as poor, ugly and stupid. In the words of Plato's dialogue:

> That being so, observe the nature of the ridiculous…. In short, it is a vice, but one that gets its name from a special disposition. In vice in general it is the part that is the exact opposite of the disposition recommended in the inscription at Delphi…. "Know thyself"….[4]

In addition, in distinguishing between two types of laughter linked with ridiculousness, Plato sets up a subdivision based on a moral judgment. Indeed, the ridiculousness observed in one's enemy is licit, legitimate, good.

In this case would it be a matter of laughter for the pure pleasure of it while he thinks that mockery combines pleasure and envy, therefore pain?

In contrast, the ridiculousness of our friends triggers a bad, unjust, little commendable kind of laughter, mixing pleasure and pain.

---

[1] Plato, *Philebus* 48-50.
[2] *Φθόνος*, translated as envy, spite, malice.
[3] Plato, *Philebus*, 48b.
[4] *Ibid.*, 48c.

In the *Republic*, Plato condemns violent laughter provoking a violent reaction in the soul and he disapproves of laughter on the part of "the guardians of the city-state" (magistrates and rulers) as well as the blessed, unquenchable laughter of the gods described by Homer.[1]

Indeed, laughter, one of the "ugly facial expressions," is indecorous, obscene, disturbing and dangerous because it implies a loss of self-control by the person overpowered by this convulsive phenomenon. It is, then, unworthy of noble, free rulers. He writes:

> Then if anyone represented persons of worth as overcome by laughter, this is inadmissible and this is much more so in the case of the gods.... Therefore, we shall not approve this passage from Homer about the gods:
>
> Quenchless then was the laughter that rose among the blessed gods,
>
> When they saw Hephaestus bustling about the mansion.[2]

Thus, for Plato laughter is a pleasure that can be generated by the perception of ridiculousness in another person. It is, then, mocking laughter, justified with regard to enemies and unjust with regard to our friends. But it is ugly, obscene, dangerous, and disruptive of society's notions of conventionality, as well as thwarting the ideals of self-control, temperance and harmony among the free people of the city-state. It is therefore unworthy of the city-state's rulers and is more in keeping with the ugliness and servitude of buffoons, lunatics, wicked people and slaves.

b) Aristotle. In the *Poetics*, Aristotle right away places the laughable and the comical in the negative camp of degradation and debasement, that of "ugliness" and vulgar, contemptible things, whether bodily, intellectual, moral, affective or societal.

Aristotle's and Plato's city-state is in fact governed by an ideal of the "beauty of the conventions and order of the appearances fashioning a common sensibility and shaping urban life," as Maurice Olender has termed it.[3]

The beauty of conventions integrates usefulness, functionality, order, the harmony of bodily forms, gestures, speech as well as that of ideas, moderation and self-mastery in all things, decency, therefore modesty.

---

[1] Plato, *Republic*, Book III 388a-389a.
[2] *Ibid.*, 388e-389a.
[3] Maurice Olender, "Priape à tort et de travers," *Nouvelle Revue de psychanalyse*, no. 43, Paris: Gallimard, 1991.

These are the values to which free people of the city-state aspire.

In contrast, excess, disorder, incompetence, lack of self-control, obscenity, indecency and disharmony, no matter what form they may take, perturb social norms and conventions. They are characteristic of peasants, boors, slaves, buffoons, lunatics, wicked people, children, even elderly persons in certain respects.

They belong to the sphere of "ugliness," dangerous for the order and harmony of the city-state.

However, Aristotle states that these forms of laughable ugliness need not be dangerous or painful, even harmful.

So they find their place within a context generating an experience of psychic and societal security in the potential laugher. As he wrote:

> The ludicrous is but one part of the ugly. The ludicrous actually consists in some defect or ugliness that causes neither pain nor destruction. An obvious example is the comic mask. It is ugly and distorted without expressing pain.[1]

In addition, comedy represents characters of a lower type, while lending dramatic form to what is ludicrous.

Finally, being one of the facial expressions of ugliness, distorting the face and causing inarticulateness, being the enemy of decency, laughter would nevertheless be uniquely human according to Aristotle.

My presentation of the main theories of laughter and the laughable will show that Plato's and Aristotle's conceptions fit into that of "feelings of superiority" on the part of the laugher and of degrading the laughable object.

B) *Two Roman thinkers: Cicero and Quintilian*

a) Cicero. It is in a passage of his work *De Oratore*[2] that Cicero's thoughts turn to laughter and the laughable. However, his reflections are particularly directed toward the laughable as produced by the orator, which he clearly distinguishes from that of buffoons and mimes.

According to him this subject consisting of "witticisms" raises five questions:

---

[1] Aristotle, *Poetics*, Chapter 5, 1449a.
[2] Marcus Tullius Cicero, *De Oratore*, Book II, 235-236.

1. What is the nature of laughter?
2. What is its source?
3. Should orators want to provoke it?
4. To what extent can they do this?
5. Into what categories can the humorous be divided?

He does not provide an answer to his first question, deferring rather to the erudition of Democritus.

Concerning laughable matters, Cicero borrows Greek conceptions, those of Aristotle in particular. Physical, intellectual, moral ugliness, human shortcomings, base, contemptible things are what trigger laughter. The entire domain of degradation and debasement is laughable.

> The subject and, so to speak, the province of laughter is always some ugliness, some deformity, for the sole means, or at least the most powerful means, of stirring up laughter is to point to and portray something shockingly ridiculous without oneself giving rise to ridicule.[1]

Orators can produce witticisms that for them constitute a social weapon that is offensive and defensive, redoubtable, effective and beneficial. This is the weapon of ridicule, an eminently aggressive and destructive social instrument, but also seductive and unifying.

This discourse on orators is, however, general in scope and later on we shall see that ridicule actually constitutes a remarkably effective social weapon, useful for attack, defense and justice.

The production of witticisms by orators is subject to a certain number of positive rules (prescriptions) and negative rules (proscriptions) circumscribing the field of their practices, which are then quite distinct from those of the specialists of laughter, buffoons and mimes.

These rules cover the themes and subjects of the witticisms, the listeners and spectators of them, as well as the use of certain techniques proper to orators and differing from those of buffoons and mimes.

Certain subjects are prohibited: misery and inordinate wickedness.

Other subjects are authorized, prescribed: human vices, bodily defects and deformities.

---

[1] *Ibid.*, 236.

Finally, Cicero discusses the two principal types of what is laughable, that of words (verbal) and that of facts (non-verbal and mixed), such as mimicry and a person's character.[1]

The jesting involving words and that involving facts are each governed by positive and negative rules.

He distinguishes between two kinds of non-verbal, mixed jesting: "Either through the relation of some anecdote the real nature of the characters of individuals is portrayed, or, through quick mimicry, some of their failings are held up to public ridicule."[2]

Orators engaging in this type of jesting must set themselves apart from mimes engaging in grotesque imitation, parody, grimaces and obscenity.[3]

The second type is represented by "wittiness of expression" or verbal humor. As Cicero explains: "Wittiness of expression is a piquant trait hidden in a word or in a thought. It is also subject to rules distinguishing it from buffoonish witticisms or trivial jabs."[4]

He then discusses "the most appropriate ways of provoking laughter."

Thus, disappointing the expectations of the listeners, making fun of other people's faults, wittily pointing to our own, ridiculing by comparisons made in jest, disguising our thoughts by use of irony, purposely letting naiveties slip out, censuring the stupidity of our adversaries–just so many means of provoking laughter.[5]

This, then, is a look at Cicero's conceptions of laughter and the laughable as applying above all to the domain of oratory, but also being general in scope.

At a later point, I shall integrate them into the framework of major theories of laughter and the laughable.

b) *Quintilian (De institution oratore, Institutes of Oratory)*[6] Quintilian finds his place within the intellectual tradition of Cicero. He thus belongs to the world of oratory. Like Cicero, Quintilian takes up laughable matters and themes, verbal, laughter's mixed non-verbal categories, certain technical

---

[1] *Ibid.*, 240-43.
[2] *Ibid.*, 243.
[3] *Ibid.*, 242.
[4] *Ibid.*, 244.
[5] *Ibid.*, 289.
[6] Quintilian, *Institutes of Oratory*, Book VI, Chapter 3 ("De Risu").

procedures contributing to breaking out in laughter, producing what is laughable and the rules governing the orator's practices as distinct from those of buffoons, jokers, mimics.

Furthermore, Quintilian inquires into the nature of laughter and its different causes, as well as expressing a certain fascination and genuine concern with respect to its magical power.

> (8)....Though laughter may seem a frivolous thing and often provoked by jokers, mimics, and even fools, it must be admitted that it has a truly imperious, irresistible power. (9) It often springs forth even in spite of ourselves and is not only expressed by the face or by the voice, but violently shakes our whole body. Moreover, it, as I said, often turns the situation around in very important matters, very often to the point of dispelling hatred and anger.[1]

Throughout Cicero's and Quintilian's discourses, generating pleasure expressed through laughter, wit or the eminently aggressive weapon of ridicule involves an obviously sadistic component that will be encountered again in other philosophical conceptions.

2. The Middle Ages. In his remarkable article on laughter in the Middle Ages,[2] Jacques Le Goff points out that this period of history dominated by the Christian tradition inherited two manners of portraying laughter. One of these, elaborated by the Fathers of the Greek Church and disseminated in the Latin Occident sees Jesus as the great model of a human being during his life on Earth. Yet, the gospels never show Jesus laughing. The other, deriving from Aristotle and transmitted to great Christian thinkers, but also to eminent XIIIth century Schoolmen, takes the opposite stand that laughter is proper to human beings (*Homo risibilis*). How in fact were the people of the Middle Ages able to reconcile two views of laughter that were so different?

According to Le Goff, the people of the Middle Ages formulated two types of discourse on laughter. On the one hand, elaborating a philosophy and a theology, they defined and judged it. On the other hand, certain of them, seeking to produce things to laugh about and to trigger laughter developed a psychology and an esthetics of laughter. Thus one finds theoretic, normative and esthetic writings.

Laughter as a bodily phenomenon also appears to Le Goff to be a cultural, therefore historical, phenomenon. It differs from society to society and within each society varies from one social group to another, but, what is more, it

---

[1] *Ibid.*, Chapter 3: 8, 9.
[2] Jacques le Goff, "Rire au Moyen Âge," *Les Cahiers du Centre de Recherches historiques,* 3, 1989.

changes from age to age. Laughter involves a combination of historical circumstances, he writes.

He then proposes readers a chronological framework for the ideological evolution of laughter that is essentially centered on the monastic milieu from the High Middle Ages up until the dawn of the Renaissance. It is therefore a matter of the laughter of a specific, well-differentiated, social group.

Thus, the High Middle Ages was the time of repressed and diabolical laughter. Establishing relationships between laughter and the body, laughter and the mouth, laughter and erotic pleasure, the makers of monastic rules developed a whole theology and ethics of the mouth underlying monastic theories of laughter. However, Le Goff detected a gap between ideology and lived reality, for the monks condemning laughter delighted in witty plays on words and compiled collections of them (*Joca Monachorum*).

A controlled liberation of laughter took place during the Central Middle Ages and a distinction was made between good and bad laughter, that is to say, between licit and illicit laughter. From that time on, there was a time for laughing and a time for crying.

Finally, during the Low Middle Ages unbridled laughter made its appearance according to Le Goff. Thus, this laughter authorized, uninhibited, even prescribed within the sociocultural context of the end of the Middle Ages would make way for the joyous, epicurean laughter of the Renaissance that we are going to look at with a great humanist of that time, François Rabelais.

3. The Renaissance with François Rabelais. With Rabelais and other humanists, laughter was ennobled, accorded new value and viewed more positively.

It would express *joie de vivre* and be inherent to sensory pleasures, thus tying in with Epicurean morality. From Aristotle, Rabelais borrowed the idea of laughter being something unique to human beings.

As a good physician and humanist, Rabelais prescribed to his readers the laughable generating pleasure and laughter, establishing it *de facto* as a therapeutic tool and instrument of mental hygiene aiming at maintaining and sustaining the health of individual and of society through procuring complex mental, sensorial and bodily pleasure.

In his *Gargantua*, he addresses himself to readers by advocating laughter in the following manner:

Reader friends who this book read,
Cast aside all passion,
And in reading it, be not offended:
It contains nothing wrong, or harmful.
True, there is little perfection here.
You will learn, except in case of laughter,
No other argument can my heart elect,
Seeing the grief that saps and consumes you,
Better it is to write of laughs than of tears,
Because laughing is proper to man.[1]

4. The XVIIth century with Descartes, Spinoza and Hobbes.

A. *René Descartes*. In *The Passions of the Soul*, Descartes proposes a physiological definition of laughter[2] and, without delving into its causes, identifies some psychological elements contributing to its occurrence.

Laughter seems to him to be one of the principal expressions of joy.

However, joy can only induce laughter if joy is moderate and when it is associated with an effect of surprise in face of what is unexpected and/or some feeling of hatred and contempt for the object of the laughter.

Mockery or derision integrates, according to him, these three psychic components and constitutes a classic form of laughableness:

> Derision or mockery is a kind of joy mingled with hatred that results from perceiving some minor flaw in a person whom one thinks deserves it. One hates this flaw and enjoys seeing it in someone who deserves it. And when this happens unexpectedly, the surprise of wonder causes one to burst into laughter, in accordance with what I said·above [article 126]·about the nature of laughter. But this flaw must be small, for if it is great, one cannot believe that the one who has it deserves it, unless one has a very bad character or bears a great deal of hatred for him.[3]

So it is that Descartes suggested hypotheses on the physiology and the psychic causes of laughter without conceptualizing them. He was part of the Greco-Roman tradition for which laughter combined pleasure and aggressiveness, the laughable falling into the category of degradation and debasement.

---

[1] François Rabelais, "Rabelais to the Reader," *Gargantua*.
[2] René Descartes, *The Passions of the Soul*, art. 124, "Laughter."
[3] *Ibid.*, article 178, "Mockery."

15

B) *Baruch Spinoza.* Like love and pleasure, laughter and jesting were for Spinoza[1] "a pure joy," which unless excessive was beneficial for human beings, their bodies and their minds.

In contrast, narrowing down to hatred or flowing out of it, joking, envy, contempt, anger were evils.

He identified laughter, manifestation of the joy and pleasure experienced by human beings, with a sign of power of the soul and of blossoming of being, therefore with one of the modalities of "partaking in divine nature."

> The greater the joy with which we are affected, the greater the perfection to which we pass, that is to say, the more we necessarily partake of divine nature. It rests with the wise man to make use of things, and to enjoy this as much as possible...[2]

Thus, in contrast to the medieval Christian tradition, for Spinoza, both joy and laughter were in God.

C) *Thomas Hobbes* (*On Human Nature*, 11.13). Thomas Hobbes emerges as the principal author of one of the major theories of laughter, that of the laugher's feeling of superiority. However, although he formulated other ideas that are just as interesting on the subject, scholars have reduced his discussion down to the sole idea of the triumph of the laugher over the laughable object being deprecated. Let us present them.

First of all, laughter is a "distortion of the countenance" that is always a sign of joy, therefore proves to be a distinctive expression of emotions.

What are the nature and causes of this joy?

Hobbes endeavors to respond to this.

- Whatever moves one to laughter must be new and unexpected, an idea that would be partially developed and conceptualized by Kant.
- He then clearly establishes a relationship between the laugher placed in a sudden position of mastery and narcissistic triumph and the laughable object as represented by the other person's present lack of mastery or that of the laugher in the past.

---

[1] Baruch Spinoza, *Ethics*, part IV, proposition XLV.
[2] *Ibid.*, "Note."

This is how he formulates this upon concluding his reasoning:

> I may therefore conclude that the passion of laughter is nothing else but a sudden glory arising from sudden conception of some eminency in ourselves, by comparison with the infirmities of others, or with our own formerly: for men laugh at the follies of themselves past, when they come suddenly to remembrance, except they bring with them any present dishonour. [1]

- He also discusses the manifest aggressiveness of laughter and the ridicule associated with the feeling of triumph, as well as the legitimate reactions of anger on the part of the people ridiculed, wounded.

> men take it heinously to be laughed at or derided, that is, triumphed over. Laughter without offence, must be at absurdities and infirmities abstracted from persons, and where all the company may laugh together.[2]

- Finally, after having presented his ideas about laughter and the laughable marked by mastery and the narcissistic sense of triumph of the laugher combined with aggressiveness toward the laughable object, after the fashion of Descartes and Spinoza, he casts a quite negative moral judgment on mockery or derision.

5. The XVIIIth century with Voltaire and Kant.

A) *Voltaire (Philosophical Dictionary)*

Voltaire associated laughter with "gay" joy and, in fact, like most thinkers, the facio-vocal expression of this pleasant emotion. He denied any underlying aggressiveness or narcissistic sense of triumph on the part of the laugher and maintained a positive, partial conception resembling that of the humanists of the Renaissance.

> Man is the only animal that weeps and that laughs. Just as we only weep about what distresses us, we only laugh about what cheers us up. Thinkers have claimed that laughter is born of pride, and that we believe ourselves superior to that about which we laugh.... Those who laugh feel a gay joy at that time, without having any other sentiment.[3]

B) *Immanuel Kant.* Traditionally figuring among the representatives of the intellectualist theories (contrast theory), a close reading of Kant's text on

---

[1] Thomas Hobbes, *On Human Nature*, 11,13.
[2] *Ibid.*
[3] François Marie Arouet Voltaire, "Laughter," *Philosophical Dictionary*.

joking and laughter in the *Critique of Judgement*[1] indicates a much richer, complex reflection.

Indeed, he establishes a sort of associative chain between the following terms: play of ideas or jesting/dynamogeny of bodily life/laughter/feeling of healthiness or physical well-being, pleasure (sensation or psycho-sensorial state).

Jesting, a facet of the laughable and play of mental representations, would generate pleasure after having triggered bodily dynamogeny or an intensification of the feeling of health, of which a burst of laughter would be a major expression that then induces an experience of pleasure on both the level of the mind and that of the body.

However, how might this game of mental representations act on the life of the body? He suggests the existence of a harmony and a synergy between the mind and the body. The bodily game would "mimic" the play of the mind on the visceromotor level.

But that play of ideas that is jesting consists in an abrupt change of the mental representations linked to the perception of something absurd and suddenly unexpected.

The mind was expecting something of a quite particular kind with the psychic tension that involves and it is suddenly presented with something else, something incongruous, absurd, disappointing its expectations. The abrupt easing of the situation follows the tensed state. This change has bodily repercussions.

> In jesting… the play begins with thoughts which, on the whole, when they tend to be expressed sensorily, also set the body into action. And while, not discovering what it expected in this presentation, the Understanding suddenly slackens, one feels the effect of this slackening in the body in the oscillation of the organs, which succeeds in restoring their equilibrium and which has a beneficial influence upon one's health.
> There must be something absurd in everything that is to provoke a lively burst of laughter (in which, therefore, the Understanding can find no pleasure). Laughter is an affection resulting from a strained expectation being suddenly reduced to nothing.[2]

Finally, adhering to the humanist conception of laughter, Kant attributes therapeutic, salutary value to it.

---

[1] Immanuel Kant, *Critique of Judgement*, §54, "Remark."
[2] *Ibid.*

6. The XIXth century with Schopenhauer, Spencer, Bain.

A) *Arthur Schopenhauer* (*The World as Will and Representation*). Another representative of intellectualist theories, Schopenhauer accords very particular attention to laughter and the laughable. According to him, exclusively characteristic of human beings, laughter, like reason, is a pleasant state that has never been satisfactorily explained. He therefore proposes a theory that he judges to be definitive and indisputable: the theory of incongruity.

The laughable or ludicrous would consist in the inappropriateness, contradiction, discordance, incongruity suddenly observed between a concept and the real objects it suggested, between intuitive presentations and abstract presentations.

> The cause of laughter in every case is simply the sudden perception of the incongruity between a concept and the real objects which have been thought through it in some relation, and laughter itself is just the expression of this incongruity. It often occurs in this way: two or more real objects are thought through one concept, and the identity of the concept is transferred to the objects; it then becomes strikingly apparent from the entire difference of the objects in other respects, that the concept was only applicable to them from a one-sided point of view. It occurs just as often, however, that the incongruity between a single real object and the concept under which, from one point of view, it has rightly been subsumed, is suddenly felt. Now the more correct the subsumption of such objects under a concept may be from one point of view, and the greater and more glaring their incongruity with it, from another point of view, the greater is the ludicrous effect which is produced by this contrast.
>
> All laughter then is occasioned by a paradox, and therefore by unexpected subsumption, whether this is expressed in words or in actions. This, briefly stated, is the true explanation of the ludicrous.[1]

The phenomenon of laughter therefore always reveals the sudden perception of discordance between such a concept and the object it serves to represent, that is to say between what is abstract and what is intuitive.

B) *Herbert Spencer* ("The Physiology of Laughter"). Author of the principal psycho-physiological theory of laughter,[2] Spencer endeavored to understand the relationship existing between the affect of pleasure, the sudden perception of incongruity, the abrupt reduction to nothingness of a strained expectation and breaking out in laughter, a quite unique kind of facio-vocal expression associated with an affect of pleasure producing an expression of bodily well-being. In order to respond to this, he appeals to physiology.

---

[1] Arthur Schopenhauer, *The World as Will and Representation*, I, 13.
[2] Herbert Spencer, *Essays: Scientific, Political, and Speculative*, III. "The Physiology of Laughter."

He starts from the premise that any intense state of psychic tension (or nervous excitement) associated with an affect generating excessively strong feeling at a given moment has to be able to be vented, discharged through one or two of the three major classical channels–psychic, motor or visceral–in pursuit of mental balance.

What would be the psychophysiology of laughter from this perspective? It is the sudden passage from one intense psychic state to another that is much less so. Therefore, it is the abrupt, descending contrast between these two states generating "an overflow of an arrested mental excitement, which... results from descending incongruity"[1] that is going to draw off the energy surplus through laughter. As Spencer writes,

> Laughter naturally results only when consciousness is unawares transferred from great things to small–only when there is what we may call a *descending* incongruity.[2]

In contrast, an ascending incongruity does not provoke laughter.

Spencer adds that this incongruity or descending contrast is also resolved by an efflux of mental excitement towards the visceral channel, which is actually observable in laughter, facio-vocal expression accompanied by neuro-vegetal manifestations and constituting a genuine bodily phenomenon.

Let us conclude by presenting an example cited by Spencer that illustrates his psychophysiological theory:

> Sometimes anger carries off the arrested current; and so prevents laughter. An instance of this was lately furnished me by a friend who had been witnessing the feats at Franconi's [circus]. A tremendous leap had just been made by an acrobat over a number of horses. The clown, seemingly envious of this success, made ostentatious preparations for doing the like; and then, taking the preliminary run with immense energy, stopped short on reaching the first horse, and pretended to wipe some dust from its haunches. In the majority of the spectators, merriment was excited.[3]

This example could, moreover, be perfectly well be applied to Kant's theory ("a strained expectation being suddenly reduced to nothing").

C) *Alexander Bain*. Bain's rather interesting conception of laughter subtly incorporates the ideas of Hobbes, Schopenhauer and Spencer. Before presenting

---

[1] *Ibid.*
[2] *Ibid.*
[3] *Ibid.*

it in his work *The Emotions and the Will*, he makes a rather banal, and in certain ways "peculiar," inventory of the causes of laughter, which he subdivides into physical and mental.[1]

Then he discusses the theory of incongruity, which he deems unsatisfactory and limited in its applications, as well as the theory of the feeling of superiority or degrading the laughable object. Why should the present inadequacies, ugliness or baseness of other people be laughable?[2]

It is then that he proceeds to elaborate his theory by combining psychological elements (affective and cognitive) furnished by the ideas of Hobbes and Schopenhauer with the psychophysiological component of "descending incongruity" expanded upon by Spencer. Thus degrading or debasing a person or "something" customarily invested with authority and dignity inspiring respect and reverence in emotional circumstances of little intensity becomes laughable.

This respect imposed by authority requiring "a certain posture of rigid constraint," that is the maintaining of a certain psychic investment, its degradation, therefore the sudden loss of it, would on the psychophysiological level result in the phenomenon of descending incongruity leading to relief or deliverance from restraint.

> A common device for causing laughter," Bain writes, "is to make a person pass at once from an elevated to a common or degrading action.... the best mode of giving the desired relief is to plunge the venerated object into a degrading conjunction, the sight of which instantaneously liberates the mind and lets the emotions flow in their own congenial channel.
>
> The Comic, in fact starts from the serious. The dignified, solemn, and stately attributes of things require in us a certain posture of rigid constraint; and if we are suddenly relieved from this posture, the rebound of hilarity ensues." He later adds, "It is the *coerced* form of seriousness and solemnity, without the reality that gives us that stiff position, from which a contact with triviality or vulgarity relieves us to our uproarious delight....[3]

7. **Henri Bergson**. In his famous work, *Laughter: An Essay on the Meaning of the Comic*,[4] Bergson presents a general theory of the comical within the context of socio-cultural life, formulating it in several different ways and

---

[1] Alexander Bain, *The Emotions and the Will*, London: John W. Parker and Son, 1859, §37 "*The Ludicrous*. Causes of Laughter."

[2] *Ibid.*, §38 "All incongruity is not ludicrous."

[3] Alexander Bain, *The Emotions and the Will*, London: John W. Parker and Son, §39 "The Comic is the rebound from the serious."

[4] Henri Bergson, *Laughter: An Essay on the Meaning of the Comic*, London: Macmillan, 1911 (authorized translated revised by the author).

giving the different procedures for producing it, which he systematizes in the form of laws. He "follows the comic along many of its winding channels in an endeavour to discover how it percolates into a form, an attitude, or a gesture, a situation, an action, or an expression,"[1] the examples of which will be borrowed from comedy.

Let us begin by citing some passages illustrative of Bergson's ideas on the comical:

> The comic will come into being, it appears, whenever a group of men concentrate their attention on one of their number, imposing silence on their emotions and calling into play nothing but their intelligence. What, now, is the particular point on which their attention will have to be concentrated, and what will here be the function of intelligence?[2]

> The laughable element in both cases consists of a certain *mechanical inelasticity*, just where one would expect to find the wide-awake adaptability and the living pliableness of a human being.[3]

> Actual life is comedy just so far as it produces, in a natural fashion, actions of the same kind,—consequently, just so far as it forgets itself, for were it always on the alert, it would be ever-changing continuity, irrevertible progress, undivided unity.[4]

> A continual change of aspect, the irreversibility of the order of phenomena, the perfect individuality of a perfectly self-contained series: such, then, are the outward characteristics—whether real or apparent is of little moment—which distinguish the living from the merely mechanical. Let us take the counterpart of each of these: we shall obtain three processes which might be called *repetition, inversion, and reciprocal interference of series.* Now, it is easy to see that these are also the methods of light comedy, and that no others are possible…. Whether we find reciprocal interference of series, inversion, or repetition, we see that the objective is always the same—to obtain what we have called a *mechanisation* of life.[5]

> The attitudes, gestures and movements of the human body are laughable in exact proportion as that body reminds us of a mere machine.[6]

---

[1] *Ibid.*, Chapter III, "The Comic in Character," I.
[2] *Ibid.*, Chapter I, "The Comic in General," I.
[3] *Ibid.*, II.
[4] *Ibid.*, Chapter II, "The Comic Element in Situations and the Comic Element in Words," I.
[5] *Ibid.*
[6] *Ibid.*, Chapter I, "The Comic in General," IV.

[A]ll character is comic, provided we mean by character the ready-made element in our personality, that mechanical element which resembles a piece of clockwork wound up once for all and capable of working automatically.[1]

After having defined the characteristics of the comical, Bergson confers upon it an asocial quality that provokes its normalization or correction through a penalty manifested in the form of the symbolically aggressive social gesture that is laughter.[2]

Thus, according to him, any manifestations of inelasticity, automatism and lack of adaptability to society that are observable in a subject and pose a threat to social life without compromising self-preservation would be laughable.

It would be the function of laughter as a symbolic social penalty to repress them, then prevent their reappearance. It is part of the system of social control in a manner that is more or less prevalent in every society.

This rigidity is the comic, and laughter is its corrective.[3]

This discourse on laughter and the laughable forms the basis of a new conceptualization, that of a social theory, which we shall return to in Chapter IV, devoted to socio-cultural facets of laughter.

8. The theories of laughter that have become classic.

A. *Preliminary remarks*. Having reached the end of this speculative voyage, some remarks prove indispensable.

Thinkers speculating on laughter and the laughable do not in fact all respond to the same questions, which are multiple: What is laughter? How does one laugh? Who laughs? Why does one laugh? About whom, about what do people laugh? Who makes people laugh? With whom does one laugh? Where and when does one laugh? What are the individual and social functions of laughter and the laughable?

Moreover, any one question has given rise to discourses that vary in quality from one thinker to another.

---

[1] *Ibid.*, Chapter III, "The Comic in Character," I.
[2] *Ibid.*
[3] *Ibid.*, Chapter I, "The Comic in General," II.

Finally, the views of our philosophers and literary figures are not just theoretical in nature, because a great many of them have also made value judgments, be they positive or negative.

Be that as it may, the majority of our thinkers link laughter to joy and pleasure, making it a special kind of facio-vocal expression of this positive affective state or inducing it (Plato, Cicero, Quintilian, Rabelais, Descartes, Spinoza, Hobbes, Voltaire, Kant, Schopenhauer, Bain.) Laughter seems to them to be a specifically human phenomenon in the same respect reason is.

The nature of their value judgments would divide those making them into "partisans of laughter" and those disapproving it.

Among the partisans of laughter, let us cite the Romans who considered it an effective social weapon, the humanists of the Renaissance, with Rabelais, who attributed a salutary and therapeutic function to laughter, Spinoza who accorded it a mystical dimension unlike ridicule, Voltaire and Kant, as well as Bergson, for different reasons, the former physiological, the latter social.

Most of those disapproving it perceived the aggressive, sadistic dimension of laughter and mockery. We may cite Plato, who considered it a form of ugliness full of danger, for the laugher is in a position of loss of self-control.

The Fathers of the Christian Church also figure here. Descartes and Hobbes disapproved of mockery and the laughter associated with it.

Now that we have presented these preliminary remarks, let us look at the main theoretical frameworks of laughter.

B) *The main classic theories.*

Four main sets of theories endeavor to respond to the question, "Why do people laugh?"

-       the theory of the feeling of superiority and of debasing the laughable object (also called the psychological (or pessimistic theory);

-       the intellectualist theories (theories of contrast and incongruity);

-       the psychophysiological, or discharge, theory;

- Bergson's theory (the social theory).

a) The theory of the feeling of superiority and debasement of the laughable object was held by the Greeks (Plato, Aristotle), the Romans (Cicero, Quintilian), Descartes, Hobbes, Bain and is found implicitly in Bergson.

The laugher would express pleasure bound to a sudden feeling of superiority with regard to the "object" that has become laughable because debased and belittled.

All forms of physical, intellectual, moral, social "ugliness," all shortcomings found presently in other people or formerly in the laughing subject are therefore laughable, ludicrous.

b) The theory of contrast and incongruity (intellectualist theories) were essentially defended by Kant and Schopenhauer, then partially by Hobbes, Spencer, and Bain.

The subject laughs following the sudden, unexpected perception in a person, in an object or in a situation of an absurdity or a contradiction, of discordance between the two present simultaneous, abstract and concrete representations of them.

Kant particularly stressed the absurdness and abrupt change in mental representations induced by jesting, that is to say he stressed the contrast suddenly occurring between the representation expected by the consciousness and that which has unexpectedly appeared.

Laughter's dynamogenic effects on bodily life will not be taken up anew.

c) Spencer's psychophysiological theory or discharge theory. Laughter would occur after the sudden passage from an intense mental state to another one which is much less so, therefore, when a situation, a fact produces an abrupt descending contrast. This then generates an "overflow of energy" blocked on the psychic plane, the surplus of which is discharged through the facio-respiratory behavioral channel of laughter.

This idea of discharge or relaxation is also used by Bain.

Nevertheless, in explaining the process of discharge, Spencer neither discussed the affect of pleasure linked to laughing, nor the uniqueness of that way of releasing energy which is laughter.

However, he deserves credit for having envisaged laughter as a process of discharge fulfilling a "homeostatic" function, which would be taken up again by Sigmund Freud in his economics of laughter.[1]

d) Bergson's theory seems to me to partake of the theory of the feeling of superiority and of debasement of the laughable object by drawing attention to rigidities, automatism and lack of adaptability to society, marks of the comical and referring to the ugliness in the theories of our thinkers of Antiquity, as well as to the inadequacies mentioned by Hobbes.

However, he placed emphasis on laughter as a social gesture penalizing and correcting the inelasticity, automatism and inabilities to adapt threatening harmonious social life.

Thus, by situating laughter within its natural setting, which is the social and cultural life of any group, Bergson confers upon it a precise function, that of playing a role in social control.

It seems to me that each theory elucidates one of the facets of laughter. To begin with, it seems there is a consensus regarding the link between laughter and pleasure, joy.

Laughter is one of the specific manifestations of the affect of joy. We are, then, speaking of joyful laughter as distinct from mocking or derisive laughter. Let us state in passing that only Latin has one word to designate laughter (*risus*), while in the Bible there are two terms, *sahaq* (positive joyful laughter) and *lahaq* (mocking laughter) and for the Ancient Greeks *gelan* designated "laughter" and *katagelan* "to mock".

In addition, in certain circumstances laughter comes with an aggressive, sadistic dimension that is disapproved of and condemned by certain thinkers. It is a matter of mockery, derision, expressing another form of pleasure. The theory of the feeling of superiority situates laughter within the framework of social relationships in which the laugher's narcissism and aggressiveness assert themselves.

The theory of contrast and incongruity takes up the cognitive dimension of laughter and one of its mechanisms.

The theory of discharge deals with its "psychophysiological" process.

---

[1] Sigmund Freud, *Jokes and their Relation to the Unconscious*, London: Routledge and Kegan Paul, 1960, pp. 148-49.

Finally, Bergson's theory, as well as those of the thinkers of Antiquity (Plato, Aristotle, Cicero, Quintilian) confers a social dimension upon laughter, localizing it within its natural setting, that is to say social and cultural life. Laughter would have multiple functions, among them that of imposing a symbolic penalty on deviance and rigidity, thus acting as a mechanism of "social control."

So, all these theories are neither contradictory nor divergent, but rather complement one another perfectly, each one endeavoring to explore one of the multiple facets of laughter, thereby disclosing its eloquent complexity and charm.

By way of conclusion of this philosophical itinerary, I would like to suggest meditating on a passage from *Genesis*: [1]

Chapter XVII

Verse 15: And God said unto Abraham: "As for your wife Sarai, you shall not call her Sarai, but her name shall be Sarah.

16: I will bless her; indeed I will give you a son by her. I will bless her so that she shall give rise to nations; rulers of peoples shall issue from her."

17: Abraham threw himself on his face and laughed, as he said to himself: "Can a child be born to a man a hundred years old, or can Sarah bear a child at ninety?"

18: And Abraham said to God: "Oh that Ishmael might live by your favor!"

19: God said, "Nevertheless, Sarah your wife shall bear you a son, and you shall name him Isaac; and I will maintain My covenant with him an everlasting covenant for his offspring to come...."

21: But My covenant I will maintain with Isaac, whom Sarah shall bear unto thee at this season next year."

22: And when He was done speaking with him, God was gone from Abraham....

---

[1] "Genesis," *Tanakh, A New Translation of the Holy Scriptures According to the Traditional Hebrew Text*, Jerusalem: The Jewish Publication Society.

Chapter XVIII

Verse 11: Now Abraham and Sarah were old, advanced in years; Sarah had stopped having the periods of women.

12: And Sarah laughed to herself, saying: "Now that I am withered, am I to have enjoyment– with my husband so old?"

13: Then the Lord said to Abraham, "Why did Sarah laugh, saying: 'Shall I in truth bear a child, old as I am?'

14: Is anything too wondrous for the Lord? I will return to you at this time next year, and Sarah shall have a son."

15: Sarah lied, saying: "I did not laugh," for she was frightened. But He replied, "You did laugh."

Chapter XXI

Verse 1: The Lord took note of Sarah as He had promised, and the Lord did for Sarah as He had spoken.

2: Sarah conceived, and bore a son to Abraham in his old age, at the set time of which God had spoken.

3: Abraham gave his newborn son, whom Sarah had borne him, the name of Isaac.

4: And when his son Isaac was eight days old, Abraham circumcised him, as God had commanded him.

5: Now Abraham was a hundred years old, when his son Isaac was born to him.

6: Sarah said: "God hath made laughter for me; everyone who hears will laugh with me."

7: And she added: "Who would have said to Abraham that Sarah would suckle children! Yet I have borne a son in his old age."

Chapter II

ETHOLOGICAL FACETS

I.   Introduction

"Laughter," Charles Darwin said, "seems to be the expression of mere joy or of happiness."[1]

Like Darwin, psychologists and ethologists agree on placing laughter into the category of emotional facial expressions, where it would "represent" joy while the other basic emotions habitually distinguished since Woodworth and Schlosberg[2] are sadness, fear, disgust, anger, surprise.

The majority of researchers hold that, like emotional facial expressions as a whole, laughter is universal and seems to appertain to a "genetically determined central motor program" (instinctive behavior or phylogenetic adaptation according to Irenäus Eibl-Eibesfeldt)[3] developed recently in the course of the evolution of the species (phylogenesis).

Here is what that great specialist of the expression of emotions Paul Ekman has said:

> If one admits that a program exists on the level of the central nervous system that establishes a connection between the specific emotions and corresponding facial muscular movements, it is conceivable that the conditions of triggering emotions, that is to say, the events that activate the program, are largely determined by the variable cultural and social learning experiences, but that the muscular movements associated with a particular emotion are governed by the program so long as the rules of expression do not create any interference and are universal.[4]

---

[1] Charles Darwin, "Joy, High Spirits, Love, Tender Feelings, Devotion," *The Expression of the Emotions in Man and Animals*, Oxford: Oxford University Press, 1998, Chapter VIII, p. 195.
[2] Robert Sessions Woodworth and Harold Schlosberg, *Experimental Psychology*, New York: Holt, Rinehart and Winston, 2nd edition, 1954.
[3] Irenäus Eibl-Eibesfeldt, *Der vorprogrammierte Mensch: Das Ererbte als bestimmender Faktor im mesnchlichen Verhalten*, Vienna: Fritz Molden Verlag, 1973.
[4] Paul Ekman, "L'expression des emotions," *La Recherche* 117, 1980, pp. 1408-15.

Moreover, the instinctive motor coordination that is laughter can also be conceived of as a mode of non-verbal, dual channel communication that is visual owing to the unique facial mimicry and is auditory owing to its vocalizations, using the face (affect display system) to transmit messages of an affective nature (joy, pleasure, but also "masked" aggressiveness, anxiety) to one's fellows. It constitutes, then, one of the many tools placed at the disposition of any subject seeking "mental and behavioral" equilibrium (Jacques Cosnier's psychic and behavioral homeostasis).[1]

II.   The Phenomenology of Laughter

1. **The "motor pattern."** Laughter possesses a basic universal "motor pattern" (a genetic and phylogenetic legacy) subject to variations that are both individual, stable (each laugher's style) and fluctuating (in terms of the stimulating situations, the subject's psycho-affective state and social context), but also cultural, explicable therefore by the intervening of a bodily technique conferring upon each social, ethnic group a style already acquired in childhood during the socialization process of the young.

It is composed of three parameters, the first two of which are fundamental:

*   **Facial mimicry** (in accordance with Darwin's description, which is still valid):

- mouth more or less open, showing the upper and lower teeth;

- the corners of the mouth retracted, upper lip raised and drawn back a bit;

- an elevated activation in the cheek region with a slight puffing in the cheekbone area;

- well-marked naso-labial furrow running from the wing of each nostril to the corner of the mouth;

- strengthening of the wrinkles running beneath the lower eyelid and around the eyes (crow's feet wrinkles strengthened);

- bright, sparkling eyes;

---

[1] Jacques Cosnier, J. Coulon, A. Berrendonner and C. Orecchioni, *Les voies du langage. Communications verbales, gestuelles et animales*, Paris: Dunod, 1982.

- eyebrows more or less raised.[1]

* **Vocalization** (according to the research of M. Lecoq and S. Beaucourt).[2] Laughter takes place during the expiratory period of respiration.

Vocalization can employ different vowel sounds in succession. Each laugher can change vowels from one sequence to the next.

However, we observe that each laugher possesses his or her special, personal vowels probably having a psychic meaning. Furthermore, the use of certain vowels can also be motivated by laughable facts and situations interacting with the subject's psycho-affective experience.

The French vowel "A" would suggest laughter full of joy and narcissistic triumph, while the French "O" would rather suggest laughter triggered by surprise, the unexpected, the sudden perception of incongruity. In children, the French "I" and the French "É" in adolescents and adults would be inherent to the pleasure of ridicule combining the pleasure of mastery and perverse pleasure.

According to Lecoq and Beaucourt, the phonation of laughter is discontinuous, sequential, irregular, its melodiousness variable, unstable, unforeseeable. It uses the middle vocal register and that of the head. The fundamental frequencies grow more and more acute the more the laughter is more forced. While intensity is variable, timbre constitutes a quite stable acoustic parameter because it is individualized.

Determined as they are by parameters of an individual, contextual, socio-cultural nature, accompanying bodily postures and gestures vary.

2. A brief typology of different kinds of laughter (according to the research of van Hooff, Blurton Jones[3] and the reflections of Smadja)

- A distinction is made between two kinds of silent laughter:

  in children, mouth open wide, upper and lower teeth showing (play face of primates);

---

[1] *Op. cit.*, Darwin, pp. 203-05.
[2] M. Lecoq, S. Beaucourt, E. J. V. Smadja, *La voix et le rire*, Cahiers d'ORL, Journées de Montpellier, June 1991.
[3] Nicholas Blurton Jones (ed.), *Ethological Studies of Child Behaviour*, Cambridge: Cambridge University Press, 1972.

the "nasal" laugh, non-vocalized, the mouth may be slightly open, associated with a slight retraction of the corners of the mouth accompanied by small saccadic, non-vocalized nasal expirations.

- Laughter especially expressed by non-externalized "internal vocalizations," without opening the mouth. This is laughter without mimicry, audible with small nasal expirations.

- Vocalized smile involves slight opening of the mouth, associated with a moderate retraction of the corners of the lips accompanied by small vocalizations.

- Laughter of medium intensity involves opening of the mouth, retracting of the corners of the lips, exposing of the teeth, vocalizations, the laugher's head being in an upright position.

- "Explosive" laughter, or the wide-mouth laugh, most often observed during children's games, involves wide opening of the mouth with retraction of the corners of the lips, "noisy" vocalizations and the head thrown back bringing about a loss of visual contact with the partner in the game.

- A "fit of laughter" describes laughter that may be intense, explosive, but is above all sustained, uncontrollable and uncontrolled by the subject.

III. **The Ontogenesis of Laughter**

1. **Problems of the ontogenesis of laughter.**

The ontogenesis of laughter raises the problem of the development of an instinctive behavior (the phylogenetic adaptation of ethologists), that is to say, of a genetically programmed behavior manifesting itself "perfectly and completely" on the phenotypical level from the time of its emergence and possessing an underlying dual (internal-external) determinism.

So, it is appropriate to envision two categories characteristic of its development:

- the behavioral structure or motor pattern.

- the dual determinism, internal or external. The internal factors integrate the neurological, cognitive and psycho-affective elements. The external factors concern the stimuli-triggers producing laughter.

It is furthermore a matter of evaluating the role and significance of the maturation and experience factors in the evolution of the two categories cited above.

2. **About the "basal" behavioral configuration.** The prerequisite for starting to laugh for the first time is sufficient "triaxial" cerebral, neurosensory and neuromuscular maturity.

- Cerebral maturity presupposes a certain degree of growth and differentiation of the nervous structures enabling the setting up and implementation of the genetically determined "central motor program," which could be conceived of as the cabling of neuronal circuits integrating several topographically defined and delimited populations of neurons within which electrical impulses and chemical information mediated by neuro-transmitters circulate.
- The infant's neurosensory equipment is operative at a fairly early stage (sight, hearing, touch, in particular).
- On the neuromuscular level, Harriet Oster and Paul Ekman have affirmed that facial musculature is complete and functional from the time of birth and that at very early age young children can emit facial expressions resembling those of adults.[1]

The process of maturation takes place during the prenatal and early postnatal periods, enabling the expression of the motor pattern, whose morphology evolves little, but through the acquisition of a corporeal technique, experience will shape laughter in a manner reflecting the specific socio-cultural group to which the child belongs.

Cognitive and psycho-affective maturation will work together, interact with the different categories of stimuli in order to determine a certain profile of the development of laughter punctuated by stages characterized by the operational predominance of one of the categories. Experience will contribute a great deal to the evolutionary profile.

3. **First laughs.**

- Starting to laugh for the first time can be situated between the age of two to four months.

The variations in timing may be a function of the earliness or lateness of the child's psycho-affective and cognitive maturity, the richness of the stimuli

---

[1] Paul Ekman and Harriet Oster, "Facial Expressions of Emotion," *Annual Review of Psychology* 30, 1979, pp. 527-54.

of the family environment, the frequency of playful interaction with familiar partners immersed in an atmosphere of security.

The laughter, often immediate, or occurring after a short lag of time, is intense. Its "automatic" uncontrolled nature and its great intensity right from the beginning (cf. the wide mouth laugh of the typology) will evolve with cognitive and psycho-affective maturation, on the one hand, and with socialization, on the other, to become less intense, nuanced, controlled and "willful," without nonetheless abandoning certain outbursts.

- • According to the work of Paule Aimard,[1] L. Alan Sroufe,[2] E. Waters and J. P. Wunsch,[3] the evolutionary profile of the effective and operative triggers of laughter seems to be the following:

- - During the first six months, from the age of four to six months, the tactile-motor and acoustic stimuli will be successively effective: a big kiss on the stomach, "stimulating situations" (bouncing the baby on one's knee, blowing in the face, "boxing," then jostling on the bed, rolling the baby over, pushing the baby), tickling (playful behavioral pattern of the fingers on the body), by themselves, then integrated into a ritualized game, like the French game "*la petite bête qui monte*," during the second six months especially. Aggressive-playful tickling causes a simultaneous approach-avoidance reaction, introduces incompatible phenomena of pleasure and fear, expectation and flight. So the child's reactions will depend on his or her mood, mental state, partially determined by the interaction partner (family member or not) and by the spirit of the playing. In the usual playful atmosphere, the child knows that the adult's aggressiveness will not be too much for him. The child laughs and retires within, the familiar interaction partner conferring a feeling of security.

Acoustic stimuli (5-6 months of age) are essentially vocalizations by the mother of the type "boom, boom," smacking of lips.

Around 6-7 months of age, the two types are found in association.

---

[1] Paule Aimard, *Les bébés de l'humour*, Brussels: Mardaga, 1988.
[2] L. Alan Sroufe and J. P. Wunsch, "The Development of Laughter in the First Year of Life," *Child Development* 43, 1972, pp. 1326-44.
[3] L. Alan Sroufe and E. Waters, "The Ontogenesis of Smiling and Laughter, A Perspective in the Organization of Development in Infancy," *Psychological Review*, 83, 1976, pp. 173-89.

- During the second six months, simple and complex visual stimuli (involving a note of incongruity, surprise and novelty, like the mother approaching her child wearing a mask, playfully shaking her hair, crawling on the floor, walking like a penguin, sucking from the baby's bottle), as well as the stimuli called "social" (according to Sroufe), that is to say, the ritualized games like "peek-a-boo," "*la petite bête qui monte*," or "I'm gonna get you" [1] will reveal their operational superiority over the tactile-motor and acoustic stimuli. The still possible triggering of laughter by the latter will, in particular, require elements of surprise and unpredictability within familiar repetition that has become quasi mechanical.

Among the social stimuli, each resumption of the game of "peek-a-boo" recreates the disappearance/finding again contrast, explains Paule Aimard. One pretends to separate from one another. This simulated absence creates a sometimes painful, even anxious, tension followed by relaxation through laughter. The game turns on that mild, bearable feeling of fear one inflicts upon oneself in order to laugh.

For Aimard, "I'm gonna get you" is a game of pursuit/avoidance that latently reproduces flight before the big bad wolf.

Confronted with these situations-stimuli, the baby gradually passes from a passive position to an active position, anticipating the known, familiar end of the stimulus by emitting "anticipatory laughter," seeking to reproduce it.

- In the second year, the child's activity enables him or her to create or reproduce stimulating situations triggering his or her laughter. One then finds self-stimulation. One year-old Adrien hides his eyes with his hands, then takes them away and laughs as soon as he hears: "Where is Adrien?" [2]

The child also deals more easily with incongruities and novelties owing to a more advanced cognitive level and psycho-affective development.

- In older children, the pleasure of "much" and "superego transgressions" ("icky poo") become prevalent. These children also possess a play signal function, an invitation to playful interaction also found in primates. Laughter going around in social interaction, in a

---

[1] L. Alan Sroufe, *Emotional Development: the Organization of Emotional Life in the Early Years*, Cambridge: Cambridge University Press, 1995, p. 85.
[2] *Op. cit.*, Aimard.

group, also constitutes a powerful triggering stimulus in children in particular.

-

4. **Synthetic reflections**–These situations-stimuli must fit into, be "immersed" in, a "positive," reassuring, affective atmosphere and be integrated within playful interactions with one or some familiar interaction partners (mother-child, relatives-child) creating complicity with the young. In this playful, reassuring atmosphere, the stimuli involving a mix of incongruity, novelty, fear and the familiar adapted to the child's cognitive and psycho-affective levels generate a bit of psychic tension that is released by laughter in accordance with the tension-relaxation mechanism underlying this behavior. However, the child's laughter also expresses pleasure and *joie de vivre*, a feeling of psychic security, the joy of being and interacting with his or her family, the satisfaction linked with achievements (motor achievements, for example) or superego transgressions (making a ruckus, icky poo).

While the infant's laughter is integrated into the development of the tension-relaxation system, it is also integrated into that of the pleasure-displeasure system.

Children's laughter therefore enables one to think of establishing relationships such as laughter-game, laughter-humor, laughter-incongruity, laughter-fear, laughter-security, laughter-pleasure. The laughter-game relationship will become objectified in young and adult primates.

On the whole, the physiognomy of ontogenesis observed reveals the existence of a twofold process of maturation (cerebral, neurosensory, cognitive, psycho-affective) and ongoing child-environment interaction (experience with facilitating effects), integrating both a positive, reassuring affective atmosphere, a milieu more or less rich in stimuli, and pervasive playfulness of familial interactions.

IV. **The phylogenesis of laughter**

The study of the origins and evolution of laughter requires envisioning recourse to a certain number of notions and concepts employed in ethology that enable one to understand better the status of laughter in the natural history of facial mimicry.

1. **Preliminary notions**

A) *The emergence of the facial reactions of mammals.* Facial expressions require an elaborate system of facial muscles.

In cold-blooded vertebrates (fish, amphibians, reptiles) and to a certain degree in birds, this system is still relatively simple. The facial musculature is more or less limited to the muscles controlling the opening and closing of the mouth, eyes and nose.

Ernst Huber[1] drew attention to the factors most closely linked to the sudden appearance of the true facial musculature of mammals: mastication of food with sudden specialization of the teeth, suckling the young (with the appearance of the mobility of the cheeks and lips). Facial musculature takes on the same structure in most mammals but, apart from the higher primates, the elaborate system of facial reactions has only developed in certain groups of some orders such as the carnivores (canids, felids) and the ungulates (horses). They possess, furthermore, a specialized, refined sense of vision with the acquisition of a fovea or *area centralis*. In them, the concentration of expressions in a reduced area (the face) has the advantage of facilitating its immediate perception at the usual distance of social communication. This development would especially take place in canids and primates.

From lower primates to human beings, one observes growing complexity of the facial musculature through the fractionation of the compact muscles bringing about increasingly elaborate and rich facial mimicry leading to the remarkably sophisticated "mimicry system" of human beings.

B) *Social play in primates*. Caroline Loizos[2] has described playing as a positive approach and flexible interaction oriented towards any component of the animal environment, including one's fellow creatures, with stimulation through the most accessible sensory channels.

Animals can be invited to play by a fellow creature of the same, or another, species. This type of invitation takes place through a signal of a metacommunicative kind (a signal informing about the quality of the communication that will follow) localized in the face (game mimicry). The play-signals seem very powerful, not very ambiguous and interspecific.

Social play takes up the greater part of the time not devoted to sleeping or eating. It is essentially observed among young people or between mothers and their children. The social play-signal consists in a specific mimicry called "game mimicry," or play face, corresponding to the "relaxed face-mouth opening" display (showing, or not showing, the upper and/or lower teeth) that is observed in higher primates and takes on prime importance in the phylogenesis

---

[1] Ernst Huber, *Evolution of Facial Musculature and Facial Expressions*, Oxford: Oxford University Press, 1931.
[2] Caroline Loizos, "Le comportement ludique chez les primates supérieurs," review in *L'Ethologie des primates*, Brussels: Complexe, 1978.

of human laughter. The motor schemes principally derive from those of agonistic behavior (chasing, fighting, pouncing, biting). Social play is generally considered to be a factor contributing to the socialization process within each species, also enabling the animal to learn what species it belongs to.

C) *The concept of homology.* Irenäus Eibl-Eibesfeld[1] calls "homologous" those morphological or behavioral structures that owe their similarity to a common origin, that is to say, that have a direct genetic relation through which information concerning the adaptation of the type of behavior in question is transmitted by the genome. A distinction is made between the homologies transmitted by the memory, "homologies of tradition," and "phyletic homologies," transmitted by the genome acting as information bearer.

So it is that the study of homologies enables one to determine the phylogenesis of types of behavior.

D) *The concept of ritualization.* In the course of evolution, numerous behaviors have lost their original function in animals to acquire a new one at the service of communication in accordance with the process of phyletic ritualization.[2]

These behaviors acquired morphological characteristics of expressiveness to become signals understood by fellow members of the same species and also act as triggers. They also acquired the function of channeling aggressiveness and enabling bonding between individuals.

2. **Hypothesis about the phylogenetic origins recognized by scholars as a whole.** One fairly relevant hypothesis about the phylogenetic origins of human laughter and smiling was formulated by van Hooff and those collaborating with him.[3]

Comparative data based on a certain number of studies establish that laughter has a form resembling that of the "relaxed face-open mouth display"

---

[1] *Op. cit.*, Eibl-Eibesfeld
[2] Julian Huxley, "A Discussion on Ritualization of Behavior in Animals and Man," *Philosophical Transactions of the Royal Society* 251, no. 772, December 29, 1966.
[3] J. A. R. A. M. van Hooff "A Comparative Approach to the Phylogeny of Laughter and Smiling," in *Non-verbal Communication,* R. A. Hinde (ed.), Cambridge: Cambridge University Press, 1972.

(facial mimicry) of the large primates, while that of smiling would be linked to "silent bared teeth display." It would be a matter of phenotypical homologies of the phyletic type (see illustration).

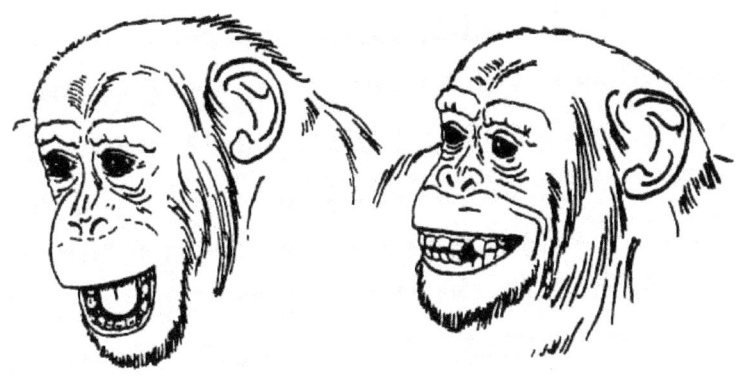

(a) Relaxed face-open mouth display; *(b)* Silent bared teeth display[1]

Thus the "relaxed face-open mouth display" would prove to be the phylogenetic precursor of human laughter and the "silent bared teeth display" that of smiling.

In fact, although appearing on a morphological level as being two expressive forms of different intensity according to the classical tradition, laughter and smiling have a different phylogenetic origin and are responses to qualitatively different motivations.

According to scholars as a whole, the "relaxed face-open mouth display" can be envisioned as a ritualization of the intentional movement of biting characteristic of playing in primates in particular, enabling it to acquire a signalization function informing fellow creatures of the playful nature of the social interaction underway or coming up. The game essentially consists of fighting and "boisterous chasing."

Human laughter would appear to be the conclusion of the above-mentioned process of ritualization. Formal homologue of the "relaxed face-open mouth display," it also seems to be a functional homologue of it, according to the ethological studies of social interaction within groups of children. Indeed,

---

[1] According to J. A. R. A. M. van Hooff, 1971, source, *op. cit.*

39

laughter and games are very closely correlated in children, where laughter signals and accompanies playful interaction.

However, is it specifically observed in agonistic playful interaction as in the case in primates? Does it always retain its original aggressive motivation? Konrad Lorenz thinks so and justifies this by the morphology of mimicry (open mouth, showing of the teeth).[1]

In adults, if one "likens" the comical to a rather "agonistic" sophisticated social game or to a playful technique of symbolic aggression among one's fellow creatures, the laughter-comical relationship might constitute a homologue of the "relaxed face-open mouth display" relationship, agonistic playful interaction among primates.

Be that as it may, it is obvious that laughter and its phylogenetic precursor, the "relaxed face-open mouth," are very closely linked "phenotypically" and functionally.

3. **Elements of comparative ontogenesis in human infants and chimpanzees from observations made by Jane Van Lawick-Goodall.**[2] This "phylogenetically playful" anchoring of human laughter also seems to be confirmed by studies of comparative ontogenesis of laughter in human infants and chimpanzees. The playful interactions between mother and infant in these two species seem to begin in connection with the very same sensory modality (touch) and with identical motor schemes (tickling, in particular).

However, sensory evolution and an enrichment of situations leading to increased complexity of playful stimuli would occur in human beings, while in chimpanzees the tactile-motor stimuli would remain preponderant and take their place within numerous playful motor schemes, agonistic ones especially.

Within these first playful exchanges between mother and child, facial mimicry reactive to tactile stimuli and specific to the type of interaction and the species appears at a comparable time (11-12 weeks for chimpanzees, 12-16 weeks for human beings).

It is a matter of the "relaxed face-open mouth display," accompanied by some little, slightly vocalized saccadic expirations in chimpanzees and by the first laugh in human beings.

---

[1] Konrad Lorenz, *On Aggression*, New York: Harcourt Brace and World, 1963.
[2] Jane Van Lawick-Goodall, "Mother-Offspring Relations in Chimpanzees," in *Primate Ethology*, Desmond Morris (ed.), London: Weidenfeld and Nicolson, 1967, pp. 287-346.

Being ontogenetically part of playful interaction, this facial mimicry would remain the play signal in the older chimpanzees, while in human beings it would also signal other motivations, intentions and circumstances.

Like human children, young chimpanzees confronting these stimuli progressively pass from a passive position to an active position, inviting their mothers to begin again, or themselves starting up the game by signaling it with their specific mimicry.

On the basis of these reflections, it is completely permissible to posit the existence of an early ontogenetic homology that constitutes a compelling argument in favor of the thesis of a contextual homology (a game) adding to the behavioral homology.

Chapter III

THE CAUSALITIES OF LAUGHTER

I.   Introduction

The study of causalities considers the intervention of two categories of factors that converge in breaking out in laughter:

-   external factors or stimuli-triggers analyzable in terms of the laughable and falling within the domain of an anthropological (but also psychoanalytical) study;
-   internal factors prevailing during both the psychic and cerebral production of laughter and its motor implementation (facial, respiratory and phonatory).

The mechanisms of psychic and "cerebral" production cannot be elucidated without the data supplied by neurology, psychiatry and psychoanalysis, human experimentation obviously being prohibited on ethical grounds.

Given the disharmonious and dysfunctional clinical aspects of laughter, the field of pathology raises questions in two areas: that of laughter's physiopathology as explored by the neurological disciplines; and that of its psychopathology as suggested by psychiatry and studied in part by psychoanalysis. Pathology then emerges as especially good ground upon which to engage in physiological speculation. So in exploring the internal causalities of normal laughter we can resort to that field on heuristic grounds.

II.   The Pathology of Laughter

1. **Basic criteria of pathological forms of laughter.** For researchers as a whole, among them D. W. Black[1] and J. J. Askenasy,[2] a laugh is said to be

---

[1] D. W. Black, "Pathological laughter, a review of the literature," *Journal of Nervous and Mental Disease* 170, 1982, pp. 67-71.
[2] J. J. M. Askenasy, "The functions and dysfunctions of laughter," *Journal of General Psychology* 114, 1987, pp. 327-34.

pathological owing to the presence of one or some of the following characteristics:

-   It is much too intense and long, out of proportion in comparison with the length and intensity of the stimulus-trigger, capable in particular of conveying a sense of "inauthenticity." Normally, the intensity of laughter can be influenced by that of the stimulus as well as by the duration of the latter and a certain number of situational, social factors such as laughing in a group during a friendly meeting or a celebration.

-   It is "uncontrolled," "uncontrollable." Combined with the preceding characteristic, this is suggestive of fits of laughter.

-   It is inappropriate, occurring in a situation that is "objectively" not funny, even within a context contrary to laughter, that is to say one that may evoke pain, sadness, anger. Thus, it proves to be out of harmony with the situation and is judged "discordant."

-   There does not seem to be any reason for it. It seems unconnected to any discernible, identifiable stimulus-trigger in the setting in which it breaks out. Stimuli emanating from the psychic life of the laugher would then be present!

-   Finally, we may mention its lack of affective tonality (the emotionless quality of the laughter) reducing it to simple mimicry.

2. Neurological forms of laughter[1].

Unlike psychiatric forms of laughter, neurological forms of laughter are extremely rare. Neurologists have documented a great variety of lesional forms of laughter (pseudobulbar, hypothalamic, temporal, hemiplegic, epileptic, frontal laughter) making it possible to formulate a certain number of reflections concerning the "cerebral" production of normal laughter.

Thus, topographical data afford a glimpse into the major role played by the cerebral structures (frontal and temporal), the limbic system, the "centrencephalic" formations (thalamus, caudate and lenticular nuclei), the hypothalamus and the cerebral trunk.

---

[1] Eric Smadja, *Approche pluridisciplinaire du rire normal et des rires pathologiques*, Thesis in Medicine, Amiens, November 1990.

The physiopathological modalities would be of two kinds: a lesional discharge during a deficit syndrome and an irritation, paroxystic neuronal stimulation.

Laughter of the *cerebral trunk* (with lesions of the pyramidal tracts more or less extrapyramidal, cerebellar, and of descending reticular formation), *hemiplegic* laughter (with a lesion of the pyramidal tract and the parapyramidal tracts) and *frontal* laughter (with the switching off of the premotor cortex, prefrontal especially) would be determined by a lesional discharge, while *epileptic laughter* would be correlated with a primitive critical discharge of the lesional cortical area spreading secondarily to diverse cortico-sub-cortical, even mesencephalic, structures.

The various different centers and effector tracts (pyramidal, extrapyramidal, cerebellar) concerned being free of pathology, their connections and the respective role of each in the "cerebral" production of laughter (programming of the laughter-laughter provoking pleasure connection, motor organization, genesis of the sensation of pleasure, motor cerebral accomplishment with coordination of the different neuromuscular effectors) have been the object of numerous hypotheses in the form of physiological models, a synthesis of which I shall present later on.

3. **Psychiatric forms of laughter.**[1] The classification established by those presently writing on the subject is fairly unambiguous and subdivides these kinds of laughter into three nosographical categories.

- the laughter of schizophrenics (delirious and not);

- manic-hypomanic laughter;

- hysterical laughter.

Let us add to this list non-schizophrenic delirious and hallucinatory laughter, as well as that of congenitally mentally deficient people.

While the lesion experiments of neurological pathology have revealed the existence of special, specific centers and tracts governing the cerebral production of laughter, through the study of psychopathological issues, psychiatric pathology has drawn us into the complex psychic world of laughter. Constituting just so many modalities of "mental encoding," psychiatric pathology reveals to us the intervention of:

---

[1] Cf. the work of Dr. Eric Smadja.

- possible internal stimuli-triggers (hallucinations, delirious ideas);

- volubility of mood, with psychic and psychomotor excitation;

- a possible disconnection of the "laughter-laughter provoking pleasure programming;"

- cognitive factors;

- the probable existence of an unconscious symbolism in certain circumstances.

Moreover, psychiatric pathology constitutes an introduction to psychoanalytically oriented reflection on laughter and the laughable that will be studied further at a later point.

4. **Toxic laughter**. Toxic laughter does not occur in isolation, but is clinically classified along with toxic manic-hypomanic bouts. Here we once again then find the relational sequence combining an elated mood with psychic excitation, the facile obtaining of pleasure and its discharge in laughter questioning the nature of the underlying neurochemical processes.

In the initial phases of intoxication or inebriation, drugs such as cocaine, amphetamines, hashish, alcohol, intoxicating inhalants, in particular, can produce an overall clinical picture of mania-hypomania.

An exploration of their psycho-physiopathology could inform us about the neurochemistry of these forms of pathological laughter, which would subsequently contribute to the elucidation of the neurochemical mechanisms underlying the provoking of normal laughter. Herein lie new prospects for research!

III.   **Psychoanalytical Aspects**

1. **Introduction.** Let us enter right now into this very complex psychic world of laughter and that infinitely variable trigger represented by the laughable by taking a look at the classic psychoanalytic texts. In the first part, I have chosen to present those texts particularly oriented toward the metapsychological aspects of laughter, then, in the second part, the writings essentially involving a genetic perspective going from the psychic conditions of the first laughs of infants to laughter and playing with words by children.

Thus, I shall begin with the founding work that inaugurated this type of conceptual elaboration, *Wit and its Relation to the Unconscious*, thought

45

through, elaborated and written by the father of psychoanalysis, Sigmund Freud, in 1905.[1]

Since that date this founding text has served as a point of reference for all reflections, analyses, commentaries, critiques, hypotheses of a psychoanalytical nature.

Proceeding in chronological order, I shall then take up Freud's second text on humor (1927),[2] and then later commentaries, analyses and contributions made by Jean Bergeret[3] and Jean Guillaumin.[4]

In a second part a genetic perspective will be presented on the basis of the research of René Spitz,[5] *The First Year of Life, A Psychoanalytic Study of Normal and Deviant Development of Object Relations*, and the proceedings of a 1986 colloquium devoted to the genesis of laughter and gaiety.[6]

Then some reflections of a synthetic nature will be proposed on the basis of this conceptual material that is so rich and promising for the metapsychological and genetic comprehension of laughter and the laughable.

2. Presentation of the texts.

A) *Freud (1905; 1927)*

a) Wit and its relation to the unconscious (1905). It was in 1905 that, concurrently with *Three Essays on the Theory of Sexuality*,[7] Freud wrote this major work, which is however, at the very least atypical, marginal, within the context of his rich, fruitful work as a whole. Unlike *Three Essays* and his

---

[1] Sigmund Freud, "Wit and its Relation to the Unconscious," in *The Basic Writings of Sigmund Freud*, tr. A. A. Brill, New York: Random House, 1995, pp. 601-774, translation of *Witz und seine Beziehung zum Unbewußten*, Leipzig: Deuticke, 1905.
[2] Sigmund Freud, "Humour," *Collected Papers*, London: Hogarth Press, 1953, vol. 5, pp. 215-21. Cited here is a corrected reprint of the 1950 translation.
[3] Jean Bergeret, "Pour une métapsychologie de l'humour," *Revue française de psychanalyse* 37, 4, Paris: Presses Universitaires de France, July 1973, pp. 539-66.
[4] Jean Guillaumin, "Freud entre les deux topiques: le comique après l'humour (1927), une analyse inachevée," *Revue française de psychanalyse* 37, 4, Paris: Presses Universitaires de France, July 1973, pp. 607-54.
[5] René A. Spitz, *The First Year of Life, A Psychoanalytic Study of Normal and Deviant Development of Object Relations*, New York: International Universities Press, 1965.
[6] Centre de guidance infantile de l'Institut de puériculture de Paris, *Bonjour gaieté: la genèse du rire et de la gaité du jeune enfant*, Paris: Editions Sociales Françaises, 1987.
[7] Sigmund Freud, *Three Essays on the Theory of Sexuality*, tr. James Strachey, New York: Basic Books, 1962, translation of *Drei Abhandlungen zur Sexualtheorie*.

writings overall, *Wit* would not be amended much, and only the theme of humor would become the object of new reflections in light of more recently acquired conceptual and theoretical knowledge (1927).

This rather dense work is organized into three parts–analytic, synthetic and theoretical–in which Freud studies wit, the various different kinds of the comic and humor.

In the introduction, Freud right away presents wit as a unique psychic activity intimately interacting with other psychic occurrences and having a status and a role in the mental life of the subject that remain to be explored. He both draws attention to the fact of its social nature and rues the lack of interest it has inspired in thinkers, psychologists, aestheticians, as well as its "obvious" relegation, without giving any notable specifics, to the vast aesthetic domain represented by the comic.

So, what significant ideas may be drawn from this major work?

-    Through the various different forms it takes (wit and its witticisms, the comic, humor), the laughable is a psychic activity aiming at obtaining an increase in pleasure. Its ties with childhood, to games– of which it would constitute a refined development– and to joyous moods were discovered and explored by Freud.

-    Three factors enabled Freud to distinguish these different varieties of the laughable, of which he gives ample priority, and unjustifiably so, to wit (according it great value, devoting three quarters of the work to it): the source of the pleasure, the topical origin of the psychic activity and the social nature – or stated in other terms, the economic, topical and social aspects.

Let us consider each one of these different forms, beginning with "wittiness."

Its pleasure results from the economy of a psychic expenditure of inhibition, of repression, itself tied in particular to maintaining the repression of sexual and hostile tendencies directed towards others. This pleasure of saving is accompanied by the pleasure of the symbolic gratification of partial voyeuristic and sadistic drives that is procured by obscene and hostile witticisms. However, the techniques of wit, being based on words (condensation, double meaning) or thoughts (displacement, false logic, indirect expression, absurdity, representation through the opposition) confer another source of pleasure, that of playing with words and nonsense practiced during our childhood and fleetingly recaptured in a witticism…!

Freud observes that these technical means of wit-work are analogous to those of dream-work. They are part of the primary process, therefore, of the unconscious' system of the functioning. Indeed, for him, in "wit" a foreconscious thought would sink into unconscious elaboration to reappear in conscious perception in a peculiar manner!

This calls to mind a reflection that he had already made in his introduction in bringing up the intimate connection among all psychic phenomena. Here the connection linking the mechanisms of dreaming and wit is objectified, though in pursuit of different ends.

Wit would be comparable to compromise-formation between the pleasure of playing with words and nonsense, that of the symbolic gratification of sexual and hostile tendencies, the demands of censorship and the constraints imposed upon one's social communication, something which seems to be achieved thanks to the ambiguity of words (double meaning) and the diversity of thought-relations.

Socially speaking, this is a process requiring three parties:

- the first, witty person;

- a second person, object of the tendentious witticism, of the "aggression;"

- a third party (or public) to whom the joke is addressed and who responds to it by laughing or smiling in particular.

Figuring among the conditions for a third person or the public to break out in laughter is being "in every way so completely in psychic harmony with the first person as to possess the same inner inhibitions which the wit-work has overcome in the first person.... Every witticism thus demands its own public, and to laugh over the same witticisms is proof of absolute psychic agreement"[1] with the first party.

This condition is of great significance culturally. It opens up prospects for research into the cultural relativism of laughter and the laughable.

Let us also mention the lack of reutilization of the psychic energy suddenly liberated by the auditory perception of the forbidden idea permitting this energy to discharge itself freely through the facial-respiratory channel distinctive of laughter. It is then a matter of redirecting conscious attention by

---

[1] *Op. cit.,* Freud, "Wit and its Relation to the Unconscious," pp. 704-05.

certain subtle means, something which would allow the communication process to proceed automatically, with laughter as the result.

As for the laughter of the public, or the third party, Freud takes up and expands upon Spencer's and Bain's conceptions. This is another one of his fundamental contributions.

"Witty" laughter constitutes a process of discharge and sudden liberation of psychic energy mobilized at an earlier point by holding on to inhibitions, repression. This free energy not reutilized for other purposes is released through the behavioral, facial-respiratory channel represented by the motor pattern of laughter.

Freud would thus say that the person listening to the witticism laughs with the amount of psychic energy saved and liberated.

Let us note that the other forms of laughter ("comic" and "humorous") are supposed to result from the same principle of economy of psychic expenditure. It is the nature of the psychic expenditure that differs. Nevertheless, the laughter may vary in intensity, depending then on various different factors, among them the psycho-affective state of the laugher.

On the psychogenetic plane, Freud links witticisms to jesting (wordplay and nonsense endowed with meaning), then to children's playing with words and absurd thoughts.

Thus, wit is an attempt to replace the playful humor of the child by rediscovering sources of primal pleasure, those of playing with words and with thoughts in particular.

What about the comical?

Freud teaches us that "the source of comic pleasure lies in the comparison between two expenditures, both of which we must adjudge to the foreconscious."[1]

The comical is found in social relationships, in persons or by transposition, personification in animals, inanimate objects, situations. It can also occur by resorting to technical means essentially aiming at degrading people especially endowed with a certain amount of prestige, power, protected by internal or external inhibitions. These modes of expression would be, among others, travesty, parody, caricature, unmasking.

---

[1] *Ibid.*, p. 750.

When the comical is found, the social process requires two persons: a first person who finds the comical and the second person in whom it is found. But if it is "provoked," it will require three parties, the third one being the third person or the laughing public.

Another essential notion introduced by Freud consists in the nature of the comical comparison, comparison between the Ego of the grown-up and that of the child, between the present and the past, left behind, overcome. Degradation also aims at infantilization.

The comic therefore offers an opportunity to engage in a comparison between two types of representation: that supplied by the comical deed depicting an earlier image of one's Self or the other person, linked to childhood; and one's present image accompanied by a feeling of intellectual, affective and/or motor mastery. This comic comparison creating a difference of psychic expenditure would be discharged through laughter. This comic feeling, an awakening of the infantile state, recovering of one's lost childish laughter, requires favorable conditions, such as that of a playful mood, expecting something comical, while concurrent intellectual activity would be disturbing.

Another important fact would be the not very objective, essentially subjective, aspect of the comic feeling. The work of comparison suggested by social reality is nevertheless intrapsychic and subject to the influence of the psycho-affective parameters of the potential laugher.

Not studied to a very great extent in the 1905 work, humor would be taken up again in 1927 in accordance with new theoretical data (contributions of the second topic and a dynamic perspective).

b) "Humor" (1927)–In this very rich article, Freud acknowledges that in 1905 he had mainly considered humor "only from the economic point of view," its essence consisting in sparing oneself the feelings which should arise from the situation and, with a jest, freeing oneself of the possibility of such external expressions of emotion (anger, fear, anxiety, pain, sorrow) observable in the humorist and the listener through a process of identification.

Let us take Freud's example of a criminal condemned to death led to the gallows one Monday morning saying: "Well, the week's beginning nicely."[1]

Freud states that the humorous attitude, whatever its nature, can be directed toward the person himself or herself or towards outsiders, something which connects up with the social process of the comical and of wit.

---

[1] *Op. cit.*, Freud, "Humour," p. 215.

The strong points of this text concern the "grandeur and elevation" that Freud attributes to humor, its inclusion among human defense mechanisms against suffering, its dynamic and topical aspects implying new modes of relationship between the agencies of the Ego and the Superego that engender a new attitude towards the painful reality in question.

The study of the humorous process led Freud to observe the confirmation of the genesis of the Superego out of the parental agency, but also to envision a more profound exploration of the latter.

Freud secondarily discusses humor as a defense mechanism against human suffering.

Then he seeks to elucidate the dynamic and topical aspects of the humorous attitude.

Here is the solution he proposes:

We obtain a dynamic explanation of the humorous attitude, therefore, if we assume that it consists in the humorist's having withdrawn the psychical accent from his effort and having transposed it on to his super-ego. To the super-ego, thus inflated, the ego can appear tiny and all its interests trivial; and with this new distribution of energy, it may become an easy matter for the super-ego to suppress the ego's possibilities of reacting.[1]

Thus, he retains the thesis that "in a particular situation, the subject suddenly hypercathects his super-ego and then, proceeding from it, alters the reactions of the Ego."[2]

Humor would then be the *"contribution to the comic through the agency of the super-ego."*[3]

Freud notes, in addition, that

the jest made by humour is not the essential thing. It has only the value of a preliminary. The main thing is the intention which humour carries out, whether it is acting in relation to the self or other people. It means 'Look! Here is the world, which seems so dangerous! It is nothing but a game for children – just worth making a jest about!'[4]

---

[1] *Ibid.*, p. 219.
[2] *Ibid.*, p. 220.
[3] *Ibid.*
[4] *Ibid.*, p. 221.

51

This text would be studied in much greater depth by Freud scholars than his writings on wit or varieties of the comic. It will therefore be taken up in the analysis of the other articles.

B) *Metapsychological perspectives.*

a) Jean Bergeret.[1] Jean Bergeret engaged in a metapsychological reflection on humor on the basis of Freud's writings (1905, 1927) and new concepts elaborated later on. Thus, he envisioned exploring the three classic parameters of any psychic yield, namely the topical, the economic and the dynamic, also applicable to the "humor phenomenon."

Humor is the product of a highly developed mental elaboration having many different kinds of mechanisms.

As Freud had for wit and dreams, Bergeret speaks of "humor-work" constituting a form of psychic elaboration of excitation, separating affects and representations and aiming at sparing oneself unhappiness in favor of an increase in pleasure.

This work would employ different psychic mechanisms such as displacement, condensation, over-determination and symbolization, combined with phenomena of secondary elaboration contributing to the intelligibility of the humorous message.

The classic themes of humor reaching the widest public are found at the level of the two major drives: sexuality and hostility, but the two are usually intertwined. Noteworthy is its subversive nature with the "jubilant" challenging of the establishment.

Bergeret then likens humor to compromise-formation and inquires into its kinship with two other psychic products: sublimation and fantasy. In the case of the latter, he thinks that humor can realize a desire in an imaginary, picturesque way just as well as can fantasies, even dreams or symptoms, on the level of latent content. Likewise, when it comes to producing them, humor is more closely related to fantasy than to wit or the comic.

With regard to sublimation, Bergeret considers humor to be rather more closely related to inhibition in terms of goal insofar as the resulting gratification

---

[1] *Op. cit.*, Bergeret.

is still obtained in the primitive sense, but in obvious forms that are attenuated and rendered acceptable.

In addition, the gratification would be accompanied by the obtaining of preliminary pleasure after the principal cathexis of the drive.

On the topical level, Freud insisted both on the importance of the foreconscious and the particular role imparted to the benevolent, protective Superego.

For his part, Bergeret considers that this Superego is, rather, suggestive of the Ego's Ideal, not yet conceptualized by Freud and actively participating in the humorous process, fundamentally regressive in nature, which leads him to reconsider humor as the contribution made to the comic by the Ego's Ideal in order to satisfy the Id without disturbing the Ego, by taking the latter back to a state of infantile narcissistic omnipotence upon which the Superego could no longer play any specific role.

Freud states that the cycle of the humorous process can unfold right within the individual without either any external participation or help. Unlike wittiness, which necessarily requires a third party and object, without which it would be unfinished, this participation of the other does not contribute anything, not even an increase in pleasure.

Humor is above all engaged in for oneself, in order to refresh oneself and to find narcissistic pleasure.

Bergeret in fact recalls that for Freud humor is produced by a sensation of threat felt on the level of narcissistic integrity. It would then aim, as has already been said, at obtaining narcissistic strengthening and refreshment thanks to an inhabitual manipulation of the object.

There is also the triumph of secondary narcissism and of the pleasure principle.

On the topical level, this humorous regression must be envisioned, according to Bergeret, in the form of the classic collusion between the Ego and the Ego's Ideal leading to the glorious magnificent celebration, restorative triumph of primary narcissism.

Thus for Bergeret, humor is always dramatic in nature. The subject runs risks. The success of humor assures the success of the drive as respect for defenses and for reality.

b) Jean Guillaumin. Jean Guillaumin has noted[1] that Freud's discourse on the various forms of the comic formulated in 1905[2] does not display the clarity and mastery found in the case of wit and humor. It seems vacillating, imprecise, tentative, steeped in awkwardness, making readers interested in the subject matter feel rather uncomfortable.

But then when Freud took up the problem of humor alone in 1927, reconsidered it in accordance with a new theoretical model, the treatment of the problem of wit and the comic remained incomplete.

> It may be thought, Guillaumin suggests, that it was the entire treatment of the problem of jesting and laughter that did not get off to a proper start in 1905.

So, Guillaumin proposes to envision this category of the comical in light of the second topic and the final theory of drives, therefore, from a new conceptual perspective, to identify a certain number of its common characteristics, no matter what form it takes, as well as to provide an account of the differences. Within this project, he has proposed a list of five common characteristics identifiable in all cases and all forms of the comical. Let us look at them one by one.

> 1. The comical, according to Guillaumin, cannot be considered to be an objective characteristic attached to a concrete situation. It is a psychic event located in the person enjoying it. Objective situations, or types of discourse, exist having a particular power to induce a comical effect. But that is only a matter of circumstances or statistical frequency that only provide an external explanation and fail to yield an in-depth understanding of the comic phenomenon, which is always dependent on the manner in which the stimuli of the situations observed or the remarks heard are received. It is rather at this level that its genesis must be studied and its nature investigated.

This point calls for some comment. In fact, situating the comical within the individual enjoying it seems completely innovative within the context of a study of the nature of this phenomenon. We have instead grown accustomed to locating it outside the laughing subject, to inventorying "classical" techniques and "invariant" themes having been the object of reflections by philosophers like Henri Bergson, in particular. An anthropological, ethnological exploration would also situate it within a well-defined social-cultural framework with its own distinctive culturally and historically determined features.

---

[1] *Op. cit.*, Guillaumin.

[2] *Op. cit.*, Freud, "Wit and its Relation to the Unconscious," Chapter VII entitled "Wit and the various forms of the comic," pp. 730-73.

However, one of the fundamental contributions of psychoanalysis has been to confer upon the comical phenomenon the psychic dimension it was lacking and which was its due.

Moreover, Freud had already brought up this point in *Wit* when he emphasized the psychic conditions of the person listening to the witticism along with those of the spectator of the comical phenomenon.

It is then important to integrate him into this list.

2. Guillaumin's second point concerns the psychic dynamics at work in the comic process.

> For him, the comic sentiment is born out of the mishaps of a kind of participation that it seems can be summed up in the abrupt breaking off of an innocent form of gratification that is suddenly confronted with emotion-filled representation in which observers feel they are unconsciously and insidiously involved, but from which they succeed in freeing themselves immediately afterward. The psychic saving Freud talks about comes, then, from the energy that was mobilized at the time of the breaking off and that the return to a tranquil state renders useless, so much so that it is joyously expended in laughter.

It is undoubtedly not by chance that the discharge of this saving of energy is accomplished through the facial-vocal motor channel, the bodily, oral prop for identification allowing the saccadic expulsion of the previously incorporated bad comical, toxic object through the opening of the mouth and vocalizations.

3. Guillaumin's third point emphasizes the role of the drive of death and aggression constantly circulating in the comic interaction between a victim (comical object) and a persecutor (observer, the person laughing about what is comical).

He finds there the prevalence of pregenital, oral, anal, urethral-phallic phenomena and an essentially sadomasochistic object relationship, the general process being regressive.

According to him, the comical fundamentally suggests a unique treatment of the conflict between life drives and death drives that varies in form (farces, plays on words, jokes, witticisms). Laughter, effusive narcissistic mimicry proclaiming life, could be considered to be a kind of reassurance against death. And for him, sexuality, the libido, would but be a "surface" phenomenon.

4. In his fourth point, Guillaumin discusses the role of the third party in the comic process as analyzed by Freud in *Wit*. This reference to the third party (person or group) elucidates the social dimension of this comic process and

investigates its psychic role. Guillaumin then identifies the following three functions in this:

-       the third party would be the necessary guarantor of the possibility of projectively distancing oneself after the initial stage of identification;

-       the third party or the group would have the function of removing feelings of guilt through the shared complicity that, after the projective expulsion of the comical "victim," they procure from the position of "sadistic persecutor."

-       the reference to the third party could also procure for the laugher a position of liberator or third party that narcissistically increases his or her standing (a leader who would incarnate the Ideal of the collective Ego.)

Guillaumin remarks that these different functions exercise control over one another, but he considers that the most urgent and most general comes first.

5. Guillaumin's fifth point concerns the laughter that he considers to be the bodily prop of the comical. He identifies three types of gratification linked to its execution: that of the pleasure of the discharge procuring a sensation of general relaxation; that of the functional pleasure flowing from the use of this facial-vocal motor channel; and finally that of the pleasure of mastery and control, of the comical object "expelled in saccadic bursts."

Those, then, are the five common characteristics of the comical according to Jean Guillaumin. The great richness of his reflections enables us to progress in our metapsychological and genetic exploration of laughter and the laughable.

C) *The genetic perspective.*

a) *René A. Spitz. The First Year of Life, A Psychoanalytic Study of Normal and Deviant Development of Object Relations.*[1] Spitz' writings plunge us into the psychogenetic conditions of laughter. His work enables us to establish relationships among the infant's first laughs, his or her motor system, excessive psychic excitation, the building up of a rudimentary Ego and his or her oral cavity. To be more explicit, as facial mimicry, emotional expression, laughter can be considered to be another form of purposive, intentional, distinctive action accomplished by the "bodily Ego" in the name of defense and psychic mastery. It would respond to psychic excitation of positive valency

---

[1] *Op. cit.*, Spitz.

induced by external stimuli (in the first place) present within the playful mother-child dialogue and discharging itself through this facial-respiratory motor channel, in keeping with the Principle of Constancy, something which reduces strain, therefore psycho-corporeal relaxation accompanied by an experience of tranquility and pleasure.

Moreover, it is remarkable to observe that the motor pattern of laughter primarily involves the oral cavity, the cradle of perception and seat of incorporation, functions essential to the survival of the species, the significance of which is also phylogenetic in nature. Would this be pure chance? I do not think so because, as stated in chapter II, laughter also has its place in the natural history of facial mimicry, where the oral cavity plays a predominant role. However, in laughter, the opening of the oral cavity seems to serve a double purpose on the psychic plane: incorporation, or introjection, signaled by the revealing of the teeth; and expulsion, indicated by the vocalizations. The oral cavity therefore appears to be phylogenetically and ontogenetically over-determined. Moreover, an increase in complex pleasure is obtained through laughter, that of successful psychic mastery on the part of the Ego and that of discharge through motor activity, but it also expresses the triumph of the mastery of the Ego.

For Spitz and William E. Blatz, laughter, and probably smiling, may be considered to be motor mechanisms accompanying the resolution of conflicts that have kept an individual locked in a dilemma for a longer or shorter period of time. The nature of those conflicts is the critical point in physical control and other accomplishments of the Ego. Laughter is successful motor functioning in the service of the Ego.

In that case, it is therefore a matter of a certain type of laughter linked to very specific psychic conditions.

However, in child development, other types of laughter emerge in connection with the mastery of other stimulating psychic situations.

b) Hello gaiety, the genesis of laughter in young children. The XIVth Scientific Day held in Paris in 1986 under the aegis of the Centre de guidance infantile of the Institut de puériculture under the direction of Professor M. Soulé proposed to reflect on laughter and gaiety in young children, a subject that had received little attention at that point. Among those participating were Bertrand Cramer, D. Stern, L. Kreisler, F. P. Espasa, R. Puyuelo, B. Golse, in addition to the organizer, M. Soulé.

As the title indicates, the focus was on the genetic perspective on laughter and its relationship to gaiety. L. Kreisler[1] associated laughter with gaiety and the mastery drive. He pointed out that the failure, the breakdown, of bodily or intellectual mastery appears in numerous situations triggering laughter. Moreover, certain ritualized games like peek-a-boo or the French game *la petite bête qui monte* also generate outbreaks of laughter subsequent to "overflowing" positive psychic excitation liquidated through the motor channel specific to laughter. Psychic mastery is "fortunately" regained. Laughter then appears to be a facial-vocal motor tool in the service of the mastery of an overflowing, and possibly positive, psychic stimulus that is part of the Ego's stimulus shield. Engaging in it expresses and procures a pleasure becoming complex, that of the psychic mastery suddenly regained, but also that of the preliminary stimulus and, finally the pleasure of the motor function itself.

Let us now discuss M. Soulé's very entertaining talk on joy and *caca-boudin* or ordinary coprolalia.[2] In this early playing with words automatically triggering laughter in French-speaking children between the ages of three and five, Soulé observes certain characteristics of the verbal comical that are phenomenological, functional and psychodynamic in nature. Let us note the phenomenon of condensation of affects and representations, expression of the primary process having evaded censorship and penetrated the secondary foreconscious process. It testifies to the fundamental principle of economy. In "*caca-boudin*," anality is present right alongside orality in a "peaceful, surprising" way and the phallic image (black or white penis) is associated with this. Moreover, "*caca-boudin*" combines two forms of sadism, that of the anal-sadistic phase and that of the oral (cannibalistic) phase. For Soulé, the expression "*caca-boudin*" therefore possesses a certain incantatory power that enables it to conjure up the forms of anxiety that the combination of these two forms of sadism awaken. In this playing with words, we find one of the essential functions of the verbal comic, specifically, that of the psychic mastery of painful emotion by a playful technique evoking, all the same, certain elements of manic defense: the transformation of passivity into activity and the transformation of a painful emotion into a positive emotion→ a transformation into its opposite.

One comes across Ernst Kris' theses. But "*caca-boudin*" procures "complex" pleasure:

---

[1] L. Kreisler, "Notations sur le corps de l'enfant dans la gaieté, l'indifférence et la dépression," in *op. cit.*, Centre de guidance infantile de l'Institut de puériculture de Paris, *Bonjour gaieté: la genèse du rire et de la gaité du jeune enfant.*

[2] Translator's note. The talk was entitled: "Caca-boudin ou la coprolalie ordinaire: la joie assurée!" "*Caca-boudin*" was translated in chapter II as "icky poo" Taken separately "*caca*" is the child's word for feces, while *boudin* is a French sausage that may be black or white.

- that of mastering painful affects (primal anxiety associated with anality in particular) with concomitant pleasure;

- that of mastering the manipulation of words having a powerful representative value;

- that of super-ego transgression;

- that of the eroticism conferred by the obscene language rich in emotions and images.

Soulé considers that for a given child and for a given family it is a good indicator of mental health when this type of playing with words can go on. The child shows that henceforth he or she can master his or her primal fears, that he or she no longer fears their representations, that he or she is capable of telling them to another person, that he or she can regress sufficiently to rediscover a very rich, very intimate eroticism, but this time in language. The child shows that he or she is capable of engaging in wordplay about his or her own fears and emotional states and that he or she is not finally far from what Freud described in his work on humor.

3. **Some reflections of a synthetic nature**. Having reached the end of our non-exhaustive exploration of the psychoanalytical literature on laughter and the laughable, it seems that we may establish a certain number of relations between the two and some very specific terms.

A careful reading of the works of the different writers on the subject suggests the following connections:

LAUGHABLE

- Childhood (with its language, its symbolic games, its instinctual conflicts generating anxiety);
- Playful mood, gaiety;
- Failure of mastery (bodily, affective, verbal, intellectual);
- Defense mechanisms, among them manic defenses;
- Compromise-formations
- Pregenitality and the Oedipal triangle (pre-Oedipal and Oedipal fantasies);
- Aggressive drives;

While laughter suggests the following connections:

LAUGHTER

- Motor activity;
- Oral cavity;
- Anxiety;
- Mastery;
- Playful mood;
- Manic defense;
- Complex pleasure;
- Transgression;
- Narcissistic triumph;
- Life drive/death drive dialectic.

All these relationships have been directly or indirectly highlighted by writers on the subject who have somewhat favored the study of certain metapsychological (economic, dynamic, topical) or genetic aspects of various different forms of the laughable (involuntary, voluntary, verbal, non-verbal, mixed, comical, witty, humorous). Nevertheless, it is the duty of any germane, exhaustive psychoanalytical treatment of laughter and the laughable to take into consideration their genetic, economic, dynamic and topical aspects, something which will be attempted at a later stage. For my part, I shall limit myself to the modest task of a synthetic discussion of the multiple connections identified at the end of my interpretation.

The laughable may be "comical or non-comical." The non-comical laughable is related to playful moods interrelated with positive psychic subexcitation ready to be discharged. It can be objectless or related to personal success, inducing narcissistic triumph expressed by laughter's effusive facial and acoustic activity. The comical laughable is voluntary or involuntary. The involuntary comical often comes from the laughter provoking interpretation of a failure of mastery (intellectual, verbal, affective or motor) observed in another person and compared to the experience of psychic security of the potential laugher. Metapsychologically, this comparison already presupposes identifying or dis-identifying play. The laughter is that of the pleasure of mastery and narcissistic triumph over the devalued object that has become laughable. The voluntary comical, aesthetic or not, whether it takes the form of witty, humorous activity or parody, even of caricature, seems to fall into the third area between outer and inner reality, an intermediate area of experience to which the two others contribute and which constitutes a resting place for the individual engaged in this work of separation and connection between two other realities. It is the area of playing and cultural experience, the area of illusion.

As D. W. Winnicott has written,

> It is assumed here that the task of reality-acceptance is never completed, that no human being is free from the strain of relating inner and outer reality…. and that relief from this strain is provided by an intermediate area of experience… which is not challenged (arts, religion, etc.). This intermediate area is in direct continuity with the play area of the small child who is "lost" in play.[1]

It would be a matter of psychosocial activity having as a model the symbolic game of the child himself, a fantastical concoction underlain by desires, one in which one can identify certain defensive characteristics such as the transformation of a passive position into an active position, the transmutation of anxiety into pleasure (transformation into its opposite), the projection of inner dangers onto the outer world, the identification with the aggressor, as well as manifestations of manic defense – let us cite in particular the feeling of omnipotence, narcissistic triumph over the object, its manipulation, its debasement. One also finds there manifestations of the primary process underlain by a desire that would be symbolically realized on the level of the latent content, as Bergeret has stated in the case of humor.

This fundamentally playful and defensive laughter provoking activity makes a remarkable compromise, satisfying the demands of the drives of the Id, the prohibitions of the super-ego, the constraints imposed by reality bound to the necessary intelligibility of the communication of the laughter provoking message, but also to the respect for social rules, finally the Ego's need for mastery. The anxiety and psychic strain generated by the conflicts of tendencies are finally resolved and mastered. There is the triumph of the pleasure principle finding its origin "beyond the pleasure principle" in the defense and mastery of painful affects such as anxiety, connecting then with respect for the reality principle and narcissistic victory with the pleasure of mastery.

In the laughable, the pleasure of the drive remains preliminary in nature and desires are realized only on the level of latent content. Voyeuristic-exhibitionistic and sadistic drives are satisfied symbolically through the verbal language and/or mimetic-gestural representation.

This laughter provoking communication can be personal and/or interpersonal. It is found in a social setting and acts as a vehicle for a language replete with a rich motor, plastic imagery suggestive of its regressive, infantile nature, something which, as Guillaumin has emphasized, activates in the observer-listener its representative function in particular and gives rise to mechanisms of identification-introjection, then of projectiverdistancing. Let us

---

[1] Donald Woods Winnicott, *Playing and Reality*, New York: Tavistock/Routledge, 1971, p. 13.

remember that Freud insisted on the deep psychic agreement through the sharing of inhibitions and repression between the creator of the witticism and the one listening to it. Indeed, "successful" laughter provoking communication is grounded in collective interpersonal psychic agreement (the cultural and social dimension of the laughable), the sharing of defenses, of mechanisms of identification and projective distancing, the latter generating the economy of a "cathexis" that has suddenly become superfluous, free, discharging itself through laughter. The group has an important function of identification support, narcissistic reassurance and removing guilt. The economy of psychic expenditure, whether it be of an affect of displeasure generated by anxiety or cathexis, even repression, constitutes the fundamental economic principle of the laughable and is one of the agents of laughter.

As for laughter, its psychic production seems complex. Freud thought that one laughs with the amount of psychic energy previously invested and suddenly liberated. This is actually one of the economic aspects of laughter. It seems to me that he "condensed" a certain number of factors and pointed to psychic diversity of meaning.

It is a matter of a facial-respiratory motor channel liquidating psychic energy that is rather of positive valency (joyful mood) and overflowing, threatening then the inviolability of the Ego and its mastery. Motor activity is then, as in the child, a function of the Ego ("the bodily Ego") in the service of the mastery of the psychic apparatus. Laughter, the specific channel of discharge, would also be a sign of the pleasure of the psychic mastery that was threatened and fortunately regained. Later, it would also liquidate psychic energy that had been suddenly saved and previously invested in certain psychic functions such as repression. This concerns the economy of laughter.

From the perspective of the dual process of identification then projective distancing that is at work in comic communication, laughter perfectly "mimes" this dialectic with the opening of the mouth (bodily prop of identification) for introjection and projection through vocalizations, suggesting the repeated saccadic expulsion of the bad introjected object. But the opening of the mouth, revealing the teeth with vocalizations, primitive vital perceptive cavity, can also represent narcissistic expansion and omnipotent mastery in the oral, "clonic" mode, suggestive of one of the mimetic expressions of manic defense and therefore also having counter-depressive significance. Laughter can in another way signal the resolution and mastery of the conflict of tendencies, with the victory of the Ego generating narcissistic pleasure, and "of compromise," that of the "jubilant connection between the different psychic agencies."

While being pleasure of mastery and narcissistic triumph, laughter is also a sign of sadistic (oral) pleasure with the revealing of the teeth ready to bite, something which evokes the intention to bite playfully, source of the facial mimicry "relaxed face open mouth display" of higher primates that was observed during agonistic social play and became the phylogenetic precursor of human laughter.

To that, it is appropriate to compare the fundamentally aggressive tone of the laughable, whether voluntary or involuntary, that seems perfectly represented by laughter. Finally, let us mention laughter as the facial-vocal expression of the "instinctual bubbling over of life." The psychiatrist and psychoanalyst Rémy Puyuelo has compared laughing to sneezing, but it is a kind of sneezing that is both destructive and generative of social bonds owing to its remarkable contagiousness.

So it is that laughter condenses multiple psychic meanings, certain ones of which prevail depending on the circumstances provoking the laughter and the laugher's emotional state. Let us cite the economic, dynamic, manic, sexual-pregenital meanings. But laughter itself generates a primal pleasure linked to the simultaneous use of the eminently erogenous motor function and oral sphere, something that leads to its much coveted recurrence, therefore, of course, to the pursuit of the laughable. So, I consider that the form of facial-vocal communication that is laughter is not arbitrary, but rather represents or perfectly "mimics," using eloquent symbolism, the psychic state and intentions of the laugher.

IV.   **Hypotheses about producing laughter**

Let us consider the case of a laughable, comical matter coming from the sociocultural milieu and not produced by the laugher's psychic activity. From the beginning I differentiate the production itself of laughter from the concurrent and consecutive muscular and neuro-vegetative phenomena.

1. **Producing laughter**. –It is a matter of a complex process bringing in different ranges of prioritized and coordinated activities generating this remarkable behavior which is laughter. My analysis examines three fundamental stages: psychic, cerebral and motor. The latter combines the respiratory, pharyngolaryngeal, phonatory and facial muscular activities.

A) *Psychic production.* – It integrates the cognitive and psycho-affective synergetic operations. Following the perception of "neutral" external information-stimuli, a synthetic mental representation is built up that is transmuted into a pleasant, laughter provoking representation through the coordinated play of quite complex psycho-affective and cognitive operations.

On the cognitive plane, the identification of an incongruity, an absurdity combined with a surprise effect will become the object of specific treatment, the positive outcome of which will bring the representation treated victoriously to be qualified as laughable, comical.[1]

On the psycho-affective plane, already amply discussed earlier, this neutral mental representation provokes laughter within the framework of an interactive social game integrating the mechanisms of identification and projective distancing, its evocation of infantile and/or repressed representation in the observer-listener, producing economy of psychic expenditure and taking on an affect of composite pleasure (pleasure of saving, pleasure linked to the symbolic satisfaction of scopic and sadistic drives, pleasure linked to a transgression of the demands of the Superego, pleasure linked to the mastery of painful affects in particular, intellectual mastery obtained after the cognitive treatment of incongruity.)

These operations as a whole "bathe" in a basic favorable, positive mood.

B) *Cerebral production of laughter.* This comic transmutation then produces a laughter provoking cerebral stimulus, one linked therefore to an affect of pleasure that will trigger the execution of the dual program: that of the laughter provoking pleasure-laughter connection and that of the motor pattern of laughter. I would like to point out that the latter can only be realized in the presence of favorable, non-inhibiting socio-cultural conditions. In inhibiting conditions, there is total or partial prohibition of the realization of the program (interrupted or partial laughter $\rightarrow$ (total or partial facial mimicry)). Moreover, this dual program involves ongoing interaction between the cortical, frontal and temporal structures and the limbic system (Ammon's horn, the cingulate gyrus, hippocampus, septum, in particular).

Let us look at the cerebral phase of the execution of the motor program of laughter:

- -the frontal cortex with its prefrontal lobes is a structure of control and dual programming (that of the motor pattern of laughter and that of the laughter provoking pleasure-laughter connection);
- -the hypothalamic region is both the principal site of the integration of the different kinds of cortical-subcortical and bulbar information and of the synchronization of the different effectors, namely the cerebral trunk in particular. Receiving input from the cortex, it organizes its execution through other structures;

---

[1] Françoise Bariaud, *La genèse de l'humour chez le jeune enfant*, Paris: Presses Universitaires de France, 1983.

64

- -the cerebral trunk, with the presence of a "hypothetical pacemaker"[1] located in the reticular system of the brain induces and coordinates the synergic action of the different motor components of laughter realizable through the existence of multiple polysynaptic connections among all the motor nodes of the cranial pairs concerned, among them the V, VII, IX, X, XI, XII;
- -of the nerve tracts involved, let us especially note the voluntary motor, pyramidal nerve tracts, the extrapyramidal and cerebellar tracts.
- -on the neurochemical level, the study of toxic laughter, on the one hand, and experiments in the chemistry of pleasure, on the other, invite us to think that the catecholaminergic systems (dopamine and norepinephrine) are involved in laughter to a great extent.

C. *Motor and phonatory realization*. This involves several coordinated synergic activities producing facial mimicry and synchronic vocalizations.

a) Facial muscular activity. – The principal dermal muscles are:

- the zygomatic major muscle;

- the buccinator muscle;

- the risorius muscle;

- the dilator naris muscle;

- lower orbicularis oculi muscle of the eyelids (the pretarsal portion in particular).

b) Respiratory activity (according to the research of M. Lecoq, W. F. Fry and C. Rader).[2] –Laughter occurs during the expiratory period of respiration. The intercostal muscles are used to mobilize the thoracic cage more than during normal breathing. The diaphragm is pushed upward by a powerful contraction of the abdominal muscles pushing the abdominal content down.

According to Fry and Rader, laughter begins with an expiration of great amplitude followed by a pause. Then laughter is sustained by short saccadic inspirations-expirations (microcycles) that contribute to emptying the lungs

---

[1] *Op. cit.*, Askenasy.
[2] W. F. Fry, and C. Rader, "The respiratory components of mirthful laughter," *Journal of Biological Psychology* 19, 1977, pp. 39-50.

more completely of their reserves of air. Laughter ends with a deep inspiration followed by a pause.

c) *Pharyngolaryngeal activity* (according to the research of M. Lecoq).[1] In the course of laughing, the vocal cords realize rapid synchronous abduction-adduction movements of the diaphragmatic motor function. The pharyngolarynx also moves. Its movements are vertical and anteroposterior and are marked by vocalizations. They are synchronous with the velar activity composed of rapid, saccadic movements of the soft palate and the palatopharyngeal arches. Upon each new inspiration the rhino-pharynx opens.

2. **Concomitant and consecutive muscular and neuro-vegetative phenomena.**

Parallel to the muscular activity distinctive of laughter is a relaxation of the muscular territories that are not involved, such as:

- the head, which may no longer retain its vertical position and rock or be thrown back.

- the hands, which may open;

- the legs, which loosen, may oblige the laugher to sit down.

This very general loosening up may also involve the sphincter muscles. The autonomous nervous system is stimulated by laughter: accompanying neuro-vegetative phenomena (vasodilatation of the facial vessels, stimulation of lachrymal secretion, more rapid heartbeat – inherent to the activation of the sympathetic system). Then a "durable" stimulation of the parasympathetic system occurs bringing about a slowing of the heartbeat, a lowering of blood pressure, and bronchodilatation with increased pulmonary ventilation, muscular relaxation, increased motor activity and intestinal peristalsis, increased salivary secretion and gastric juices. Laughter also allows the freeing of cerebral endorphins, reducing nociceptive (painful) sensations.

Finally, by being engaged in, and through its beneficial physiological effects, laughter, the facial-vocal expression of an affect of pleasure, itself generates bodily, functional pleasure, leading then easily to its recurrence and making it one of the most powerful stimuli for provoking laughter. Thus, we observe that laughter is much more than simple facial mimicry accompanied by vocalizations. It is a total psychic, corporeal phenomenon. Common sense has traditionally held it in derision. Such an opinion is now outdated.

---

[1] *Op. cit.*, Lecoq, Chapter 11.

Having come to the end of this study of ethological, pathological, psychoanalytical and physiological approaches to laughter, the initially inextricable complexity of laughter seems to have been overcome. It is now time to leave the "laboratory" and the "hospital" where it sojourned during the time required for experimentation and research on it and reinsert it into its natural setting, which is the socio-cultural life of a group.

Chapter IV

SOCIO-CULTURAL FACETS

I.   Introduction

Looking at anthropologists' relationship to the laughter of the indigenous peoples they study, in his book *Le propre de l'homme*, Jean Duvignaud writes

> Ethnologists, anthropologists hardly speak of laughter. No doubt, they are wary of the comical and funny aspects of life together? It is true that derisiveness disturbs the coherence of systems, the internal logic of structures or the seriousness of the observers.... However, the notes taken day after day (when they are published), the conversations recorded, the photographs, the films show moments of merriment that later disappear from the study once drawn up![1]

Indeed, it definitely seems that anthropological literature, whether ethnographical or theoretical, scarcely provides any systematic studies of the laughable and laughter of societies. The laughable, the comical, humor, laughter do not seem to be considered to be "serious subjects," therefore worthy of ethnographical observation and analysis, then of theoretical treatment. Yet, they are not funny either! Categorized and misplaced in the domain of the trivia of social life, hoaxes, jokes, pranks have not really aroused the interest of ethnologists primarily concerned, and completely legitimately so, with exploring the different areas of social organization, kinship, economics, politics, ideologies and describing the material culture, something which they have undertaken with great seriousness and in an exemplary fashion.

"The study of rules, functions, mentalities, structures and their various combinations," Duvignaud writes,

> undoubtedly responds to the firm intent to define the stability, the cohesiveness and the preservation of societies. It rarely tells us how women and men accept, bear, bypass, distort these controls and prescriptions, invisible or not, that define a culture. We do not know very much about the manner in which the living live society.... In the best of cases, we are referred to what is marginal, atypical, just

---

[1] Jean Duvignaud, *Le propre de l'homme: Histoires du rire et de la dérision*, Paris: Hachette, 1985, p. 19.

so many terms used to try to conjure up what one does not understand. And that does not account for dawdling, lingering, playing, passions, the useless moments of existence.... That takes us to an unexplored region of human experience.... Do not the comical, mockery belong to this obscure, uncharted area?[1]

Indeed, "this obscure, uncharted" area of human experience represented by the laughable and laughter raises multiple questions: its delimitation within the fabric of the daily, social life of groups, its structure, its functions, its multiple, polymorphous practices governed by positive and negative rules, its culturally and historically determined representations, its possible interactions and relations with other sectors of social life in particular.

Thus we find that defining the anthropological issues surrounding the laughable and laughter proves to be perilous. Yet if we pursue the course we initially adopted, which consists of using the positive, unifying concept of communication, then as a form of facial-vocal communication emitting affective messages of pleasure, aggressiveness, anxiety (denied or not), laughter would also accord with the comical laughable understood as another quite unique form of social communication. Once this stage of reflection has been reached, some simple questions applying to any social group can be asked: Who laughs? How does one, or do they, laugh? Why do they laugh? Where and when do they laugh? About whom, about what do they laugh? With whom do they laugh? What makes people laugh? This simple, abstract questioning of all observable facts will guide our interpretation of classic ethnographic writings dealing historically and geographically with the different groups within which laughter and laughing matters have been brought up. This constitution of henceforth valuable ethnographic documents would form the basis of an analytic and synthetic reflection capable of determining the formulation of working hypotheses and thus shed light on the socio-cultural encoding of laughter.

II.   Ethnographical Facts

1. **Introduction.** –I have deliberately chosen texts recounting various different aspects of the social life of ethnic groups that mainly differ from one another in that they belong to a specific geographical area. Nevertheless, I shall particularly study those of the Americas since they have already been the object of earlier study. In the Americas, we shall look at:

---

[1] *Ibid.*, pp.14-15

- with Claude Levi-Strauss, the social and family life of the Nambikwara figuring in *Tristes Tropiques;*[1]

- with Pierre Clastres, the life of the Guayaki of Paraguay;[2]

- with Don Talayesva, the social life of the Hopi and their famous sacred clowns.[3]

In Africa, other than the study by Françoise Héritier-Augé on the laughter of African children figuring in the specialized literature, I take a look at a certain type of laughter and the laughable found by Colin Turnbull among the Ilk of northeastern Uganda within a context of tragic social change having brought about a profound disruption of the social life of a tribe and involving a major threat to their existence: famine. What exactly can one laugh about when one's survival is at stake?

2. In the Americas.

A) *The Nambikwara, a people of great interest here.*

"Whether traditional or degenerate," wrote Levi-Strauss, "this society offered one of the most rudimentary forms of social and political organization that could possibly be imagined."[4] This semi-nomad population of central Brazil lives in bands.

During the time he spent there, Levi-Strauss lived in one of these bands comprising around twenty-three members divided into six families, one of which was that of the chief (with his three wives and adolescent daughter) and five others. Each band was made up of a married couple and one or two children. Kinship bonds existed among its members and the preferred rules of marriage authorized unions with one's niece (the daughter of one's sister) or a cross-cousin. So from the time of birth, these cross-cousins are called spouses, while parallel cousins are called brothers and sisters and cannot intermarry.

---

[1] Claude Levi-Strauss, *Tristes Tropiques*, tr. John and Doreen Weightman, New York: Penguin Books, 1992.
[2] Pierre Clastres, *Chronicle of the Guayaki Indians*, tr. Paul Auster, New York: Zone Books, 1998.
[3] Don Talayesva, *Sun Chief, the Autobiography of a Hopi Indian*, New Haven: Yale University Press, 1942.
[4] *Op. cit.*, Levi-Strauss, p. 316.

A dual economy is to be found there: the men are hunters and gardeners, the women collectors and gatherers. Thus the married couple forms an economic unit and a stable reality.

The name used to designate the chief in the Nambikwara language is Uilikandé ("he who unites" or "he who joins together"). Power derives from consent and this is what maintains its legitimacy. The chief has no power of coercion. He must do well and do better that the others. The chief has power, but he must be generous. He has duties, but he can obtain many wives. Between him and the group is established a perpetually renewed balance of gifts and privileges, services and obligations.

Among his obligations and flowing from his generosity, the chief must be a good singer, a good dancer and a "jolly fellow" always ready to entertain and to make the band laugh, in this way breaking the monotony of daily life.

- The band seems to be organized into groups or micro-societies:

- that of the men, who spend their time hunting, gardening, doing basketwork, making bows and arrows, even musical instruments;

- that of the women, who spend their time mothering, cooking, collecting and gathering, as well as doing arts and crafts;

- the children remain close to their mothers until weaned, while little girls and young women each form close-knit, homogeneous groups within which connivance and complicity reign. In contrast, the boys rather seem left to their own devices not managing to form a cohesive band.

Let us not forget the domestic animals composed of dogs, cocks, hens, monkeys, parrots in particular, whose status and function within the band are fairly specific.

The fabric of daily life of this Nambikwara band seems manifestly sprinkled with, punctuated by, the laughable and laughter. So it is that they can be found as women are engaging in the household tasks or arts and crafts activities that accompany conversations interspersed with joking and bursts of laughter. "Almost always merry and gay, they make jokes or sometimes obscene or scatological remarks, which are greeted by great guffaws of laughter."[1]

---

[1] *Ibid.*, p. 281.

Mother-child relationships are marked by a certain emotional warmness allowing the establishment of playful interactions in the course of which laughter emerges. "[A] young mother was playing with her baby by giving him gentle slaps on the back; the baby started to laugh and the mother became so caught up in the game that she struck him harder and harder until he began to cry. Whereupon she stopped and consoled him."[1]

The relationships between young women and girls making up homogeneous groups also seem to be thoroughly playful. They play and joke also with the children.

The only form of amusement that boys engage in consists in wrestling matches or playing tricks on one another, or even games with domestic animals.

Adults laugh at the "future spouses" behavior on the part of the children enjoying the prescribed cousin relationship and so calling one another "husband-wife."

"In all matters concerning love," writes Levi-Strauss, "the natives show the highest degree of interest and curiosity; they are eager to talk about such subjects and their conversation in the encampment is full of allusions and innuendoes."[2]

Let me also point out the amorous play that couples indulge in publicly, triggering bursts of laughter.

Finally, let me mention the way the Nambikwara live in very close association with their domestic animals that are themselves treated like children, receiving the same marks of affection, caresses, delousing too. While the dogs have a utilitarian function in hunting with sticks, cocks, hens, monkeys, parrots are raised for the pleasure they bring. They provide the group with a source of entertainment, amusement, the laughable and laughter.

Thus, for the Nambikwara, the laughable is a daily affair, does not seem fabricated, "aesthetic;" it can be voluntary or involuntary. The job of the chief, a jolly person, and of the domestic animals is, among other functions, to entertain the group, to make them laugh. The playful context is the preferred spatiotemporal social setting for producing and spreading the laughable and laughter. The times of relaxation and reestablishing the unity of the group are so too. The laughable and laughter combine psychic security with conviviality and social complicity. Sexuality proves to be a central, predominant theme of

---

[1] *Ibid.*, pp. 282-83.
[2] *Ibid.*, p. 285.

"laughter-provoking messages." I did not find in Levi-Strauss' writings any rules concerning the expression of laugher, or any bodily technique for it.

On the basis of these facts, would it be pertinent to envision relationships existing between the forms of the laughable and laughter and the meagerness of the social, political, economic organization, or even the rudimentary nature of their material culture?

Before contemplating this question, let us look at the facts about the Guayaki gathered in Pierre Clastres' *Chronicle*.[1]

B) *The Guayaki.*

This is a population of nomadic hunters and gatherers of Paraguay living in bands of 20 to 25 people, who all come together in the same camp in June of each year for the festival of Honey. In this way the tribe restores its unity. Their social, political and economic organization shows strong analogies with that of the Nambikwara.

"A man can only think of himself as a hunter, one cannot be a man and not a hunter at the same time. The entire symbolic space of masculinity unfolds in the act.... of *lyvo*, shooting an arrow...."[2] When a man is not a hunter, the group does not take him seriously.

Women engage in collecting and gathering, the basket being one of the symbols of femininity. Thus we obtain two sets of equations:

Man = hunter = bow
Woman = gatherer = basket

The adults are very interested in sexuality. They "make no effort to hide sexuality or the subject of sexual activities from the children [*kybuchu*]. In their presence, and without any embarrassment, they discuss *meno* (making love), the adventures and experiences of various lovers, and the jokes made about these matters are understood by everyone."[3]

The *kybuchu* find it very amusing to watch the adults.

---

[1] *Op. cit.,* Clastres.
[2] *Ibid.,* pp. 279, 281.
[3] *Ibid.,* p. 202.

-       Laughing matters and laughter.

The Guayaki being as discreet about taking care of their bodies as about their love life, the *kybuchu* (children) amuse themselves at the expense of the adults, spying on them in their private activities.

Also observed were erotic caresses and games between men and women, husbands and wives, during which people engage in laughter.

Setting aside sexuality, the primary subject of laughter, psychosocial deviance with regard to the accepted, respected norms constitutes another subject of the laughable and laughter, both in children and adults. Since men are identified with hunting, women with gathering with their baskets, a man who is not a hunter and carries a basket is a deviant. He is mocked and ridiculed. Clastres encountered a person of this sort during his stay with a band of Guayaki (the Atchei Gatu).

The Atchei's festival of Honey and of the New Year (at the end of June) is the annual time for restoring tribal unity, but also the time of alliances, of exchanges of women between men of different bands, of love affairs for men and women who are already married, of playing and "hysterical" laughter. The festival has many phases:

It begins with a display of violence.

After the feigned declaration of war must come the ritual of reconciliation... a ceremonial game, the necessary prelude to all phases of the ritual, the *kyvai*: the tickling. Two by two, putting their arms around each other, the warriors run their fingers into the armpits and down the ribs of their partners. It is a sort of competition to see who will be the last to laugh. They try to hold back as long as possible and endure the tickling, which is a form of torture they are not used to. By allowing men to touch each other, the true function of *kyvai* becomes clear... to establish or strengthen friendship between two men.[1]

The *kyvai* having been engaged in, the women sing ritual greetings. The men sing of their hunting exploits, "shouting, singing, laughter, music, good food; all the friends are there, the women are beautiful.... They are so happy that they laugh. The next day they will take the *proaa*."[2] This is a kind of large bean similar to the European fava bean. In the game of *proaa mata*, a man or a woman places one of these beans under his or her armpit or in his or her fist. It is a question of forcing the person possessing the bean to give it up. The person is tickled and must give up. Then the winner triumphantly brandishes the

---

[1] *Ibid.*, pp. 226-27.
[2] *Ibid.*, p. 229.

coveted *proaa* in the air. All the adults gang up to tickle the person having the bean. So the whole time the tribe is gathered together they play at grabbing the bean. This is also an occasion for amorous encounters! The festival of Honey is the festival of the body and the annual time for pleasure, for "prescribed" breaking of taboos surrounding touching. Aggression becomes friendships. Friendships are made through "prescribed" aggression, by tickling (the ambivalent practice *par excellence*).

In concluding this presentation of laughing matters selected from my reading of the *Chronicle of the Guayaki Indians*, I shall formulate some ideas by way of synthesis: the laughable is daily, voluntary and involuntary, often being found in a playful setting and developing within a relationship that sets individuals of different ontological categories (men/women, children/adults, boys/girls-young women) up against one another. Combined with social deviancy, sexuality stands out as a central theme being the object of ridicule.

Social deviancy as a laughing matter is also a sign of belonging to a group having established behavioral schemes and social norms, as well as constituting one of the effective modes of social control.

In contrast to the Nambikwara, I identify a new spatiotemporal, socio-cultural setting "specialized" in producing and freely spreading the laughable and laughter: celebrations, high point in the life of a society, one of whose laws consists in transgressing prohibitions. The Guayaki's ban on touching, or "extra-erotic" bodily contact, is also transgressed in a remarkable manner in the form of a ceremonial game through tickling and the *proaa mata*. They display and/or strengthen friendship through aggression.

C) *The Hopi*

a) *Brief presentation that can orient intelligibility of the laughable.* The Hopi are the western representatives of the Pueblo Indians (of the American Southwest) presently living in about ten villages located in northeastern Arizona. They are divided into clans. Descent, inheritance and succession are matrilineal and residence is matrilocal. The Hopi pantheon of gods is rather complex. The Sun is the highest god. The rain-bearing clouds are identified with the ancestors. Let us especially mention the Katcinas, who themselves alone form a people of special deities that embody the supernatural companions of the first ancestors (or these ancestors themselves) and who spend six to nine months of the year in the village as masked dancers, dancing almost daily for the adults and children. They arrive in the village in December and depart in July, and the end of the Niman dance (celebration held when the Katcinas are sent home for the season).

b) Laughing matters and laughter. – Talayesva's rich autobiography may be said to contain numerous, fairly diversified laughable matters and situations. I have selected the most representative ones for the purposes of my analysis.

Thus, in childhood, we observe three categories of relationships in the course of which the laughable and laughter are present. It is a question of playful interaction between adults and children at the expense of the latter, among children and between children and animals. This type of interaction takes the concrete form of jokes, pranks and hoaxes of all kinds. Let us take a brief look at these three categories of laughter-provoking interaction.

It must be noted that the adults often tickle the sexual organs of all the male children to make them laugh and keep them from crying.

> After I was four or five nearly all my grandfathers, father's sisters' and clan sisters' husbands played very rough jokes on me, snatched at my penis, and threatened to castrate me, charging that I had been caught making love with their wives, who were my aunts. All these women took my part, called me their sweetheart, fondled my penis, and pretended to want it badly. They would say, "Throw it to me," reach out their hands as if catching it, and smack their lips. I liked to play with them but I was afraid of their rough husbands and thought they would castrate me. It was a long time before I could be sure that they meant only to tease.[1]

Among children, taunting is rampant: "At the races people teased me and said that my feet turn out so far that I pinched my anus as I ran."[2]

Games with animals and at their expense are very frequent and liven up their days; "We chased chickens, threw corncobs at them, and shot them with our toy arrows. We encouraged roosters to fight for our amusement.... We often played with dogs and cats, and sometimes we encouraged them to fight."[3]

Among adults, sexual hoaxes, jokes, pranks essentially go on more or less freely. Sexuality is a laughing matter, procuring pleasure, but it also serves to degrade another person (a man, woman, spouse, friend, stranger, deviant) and the Sacred in particular. Sexuality is subject to mockery.

Two institutionalized settings of the laughable and laughter distinctly stand out in Hopi life:

---

[1] *Op. cit.*, Talayesva, p. 40.
[2] *Ibid.,* p. 69.
[3] *Ibid.,* p. 62.

-      celebrations particularly linked to rites of passage (the *wowochim* or tribal initiation and marriage);

-      the Katcina dances and ceremonial clowns, themselves laughter institutions.

The pranks and hoaxes of the clowns that are part of the comical in Hopi life attain the sacred universe, sexuality, the various different kinds of misfortune and bad luck, men and women, outsiders (Navajos, Comanches, Paiutes, Whites), deviants, animals. They engage in mockery, using parody and the language of sexuality, among other techniques aiming at the distinct debasement of the object that has become laughable.

Don Talayesva became a clown. He wrote,

The clown work afforded a good opportunity to play jokes on people, chastise them for misbehavior, and even to take out spite on them. A clown could do or say almost anything and get away with it because his duty was sacred. Therefore we teased and joked the Christians in our clown work.[1]

Now let us leave the Americas for Africa.

3. In Africa.

A. West Africa. – In her article "Fait-on rire les enfants en Afrique?," initially the topic of a talk given during Michel Soulé's scientific day on the genesis of laughter and gaiety in young children, Françoise Héritier-Augé[2] observed on the basis of facts gathered in the literature that the laughter of African children falls into the category of certain types of culturally determined social and familial interaction.

Laughter is often perceived as an explosive display of vitality. From birth to weaning (2-3 years), young children living in the parental domain are fragile, endangered beings. They must not attract the attention and the destructive desire of malevolent powers by their laughter or by expressing themselves positively in other ways leading consequently to their early death.

Thus, laughter does not figure as a positive signal in parent-child interactions. Moreover, Héritier-Augé points out that in African societies this

---

[1] *Ibid.*, p. 280.
[2] Françoise Héritier-Augé, "Fait-on rire les enfants en Afrique," Centre de guidance infantile de l'Institut de puériculture de Paris, *Bonjour gaieté: la genèse du rire et de la gaité du jeune enfant*, Paris: Editions Sociales Françaises, 1987.

type of relationship (parent-child) is characterized by respect and distance, unlike relations between alternate generations (grandparents and grandchildren) or within the same age group and within the same generation where, however, seniority implies respect.

It is then that we observe playful, joyful interaction between grandparents and their grandchildren during which laughter bursts out, however, less frequently so, it seems, than bodily contact, caresses and verbal exchanges. This interrelational distance between parents and children may be explained by the fact that a child is very generally not considered to be new being. In a certain way he or she is, Héritier-Augé explains, an ancestor who has chosen to come back in this child or who has been forced to do so. He or she is owed deference. One must already act in such a way that he or she remains. Those who come back may find that the existence being proposed to them is not to their liking. When children die young, this is thought to be due to this reticence to live through a reincarnated ancestor or through a part of him or her that has come back in this child.

Thus certain forms of distant, deferential, attentive parental behavior towards children may be explained by the fact that the baby is an ancestor.

By the age of 3-4 years, the children have left the parental domain to enter into the community of children (age group) where two sorts of social interaction prevail: playing and laughing, but also educational.

Indeed, the children play together, engage in friendly quarreling, but also joke, play pranks on one another. When it comes to upbringing, the age group gives children an opportunity to learn the rules of etiquette and good manners, along with learning social practices favored by their parents. It is then an eminently important place for the child's socialization as well as for exercising social control, in particular through mockery and ridicule. Héritier-Augé's most interesting article particularly shows the advantage of being able to identify certain forms of social and familial interaction–one of the parties to which is the child–authorizing, prescribing or prohibiting the production and spreading of the laughable and laughter in West African societies. In addition, it furnishes certain conceptual tools making it possible to document some of the functions and meanings inherent in these practices.

B) *Laughter and laughing matters among the Iks.* Calling themselves the "*Kwarikik*," that is the people of the mountain, the Iks make up an ethnic group of nomadic hunters and gatherers organized into bands who, just prior to World War II, settled in the mountainous region in northeastern Uganda. The Kidepo Valley at the foot of Mount Morungole (the Iks' sacred mountain) was their principal hunting ground.

However, the decision of the Ugandan government to create a natural park, the Kidepo Valley National Park, part of the Iks' economic territory, forced their eviction, obliging them to settle down elsewhere and to practice "agriculture" in an poor, arid region in order to "make up for the lack of resources."

During his stay there between 1965 and 1967, Colin Turnbull[1] was able to observe the extent of the socio-economic tragedy experienced by this traumatized population, which manifested itself in a profound deterioration of family and social ties, combined with distrust, individualism, hetero-aggressiveness, extreme impoverishment, even a loss of all religious and ritual life, physical decline especially affecting the children and the elderly, all of these disruptions of their life inseparable from the tragic famine.

The Iks' social existence had from that time been essentially organized around a frenetic search for food and the development of a new system of values in which procuring food and adapting to these precarious conditions of survival played the primary role. Within this intensely painful life and social context, to his great surprise, Turnbull found much laughter and many situations that made the Iks laugh. Among the laughter-provoking subjects figured hunger, kindness, generosity (deviant qualities), the decline and suffering of others, even one's own, in certain circumstances, the behavior of strangers (Dodo and Turkana neighboring tribes, cattle-herders with whom the Iks do business and exchange goods and services). Communication through laughter could take place among young people, adults, men, women, the elderly, be engaged in at the expense of those who were weak (children, the elderly), women, those considered deviants by the group, outsiders.

With Turnbull, let us look at certain examples of laughter and laughable matters that are rather surprising for us, but fulfill functions and have meanings that remain to be discovered.

On the subject of hunger and physical decline:

I said goodbye to the two men and got up to leave, but as I did a strange thing happened. I was shaking hands with the older man and as I moved to take my hand away he tightened his grip so that I found myself actually pulling the old man off the ground. I don't think he could have weighed more than sixty pounds.... his grip weakened... and he fell back and collapsed and lay on the ground... and he was laughing. He held out his hand, still laughing breathlessly, for me to help him back to a sitting position. He apologized for his behavior. "I

[1] Colin M. Turnbull, *The Mountain People*, New York: Simon & Schuster, 1972.

haven't eaten for three days"... he and his companion dissolved into laughter. I felt there was going to be much I had to learn about Ik humor.[1]

The laughter of a mother at the expense of her child who is hurt:

> in the process of being cared for he or she is carried about in hide sling wherever the mother goes.... Whenever the mother finds a spot in which to gather, or if she is at a water hole or in her fields, she loosens the sling and lets the baby to the ground none too slowly, and of course laughs if it is hurt. I have seen... this many a time.[2]

The laughter of children at the expense of old people:

> Once again I found him [Lolim an elderly ritual priest] with Lokwam and a gang of children around him shouting and throwing little stones at him... and Lolim was rolled up in his protective ball....[3]

What then is one to think of this laughter in this profoundly disorganized tragic socio-cultural context? It could be a sign of the inherent pleasure a person feels in continuing to adapt to harsh, painful existential conditions in comparison to the failure and incompetence observed in another person, in young children and the elderly in particular. It is then a matter of "triumphant mastery" of a painful situation and of the security conferred by continuing, though constantly endangered, narcissistic wholeness. But this laughter can also be a defense against death and object loss anxiety, a form of denial of ongoing danger to one's life and reassurance against this danger. In face of human decline, the ever greater reality of death and the ongoing danger of it to which the Iks, especially the children, were exposed, laughter triumphantly affirms life and is an attempt to deny death. Mocking the decline of the elderly can be a form of protection against the painful affects inherent in it. Laughter and mockery would then constitute a psychosocial tool of psychic survival in the Iks. And contrary to all predictions, in 1987, after twenty years of suffering, the Iks were surviving. Despite the terrible famine observed by Turnbull in 1965, despite a cholera epidemic in 1973-1975 and additional years of want, they managed to maintain a population of between 1,000 and 2,000 people. Life among the Iks is stronger. Might laughter and mockery have contributed to the psychic survival of this ethnic group in danger of dying out?

---

[1] *Ibid.*, p. 49.
[2] *Ibid.*, p. 135.
[3] *Ibid.*, p. 206.

III. Presentation of the "Laughable-Laughter" Communication System

1. **Introduction.** The ethnographic facts discussed above have inspired a certain number of reflections and questions, as well as having acquired the status of being valid "ethnographic documents," thus contributing to the constitution of a body of knowledge relative to a new field of anthropological studies, that of the laughable and laughter. This research consisting in the methodological and conceptual organization of the field has been pursued through the reading and consultation of other anthropological–but also sociological, psycho-sociological, historical, literary–writings structuring and enriching my intellectual undertaking. So my working hypothesis only represents one mode of socio-cultural approach to laughter and the laughable laying down the theoretical bases for work in the field.

Studying it within the social life of a group, my approach establishes laughter as a cultural, therefore historical, cultural phenomenon. It is of all times and in all places. People neither laugh in the same way, nor at the same things, from one society to another or from one era to another. Each society creates its laughter and what it considers laughable. However, despite the cultural variants, the presentation of ethnographical facts has also made it possible to identify characteristics of laughter and the laughable that do not vary from one culture to another.

2. **"Laughable-Laughter" Communication**. Since laughter is very probably a matter of an encoded bodily technique, for purposes of cultural intelligibility, it may also be viewed as one of the elements of a unique form of social communication called a laughable communication system. To present and describe it, I have been inspired by the schematic diagram of communication worked out by Claude Shannon and Warren Weaver.[1] Situated in the third area defined by D. W. Winnicott, psychoanalyst, this form of social communication would have two poles: a psychic/elaborative pole and a phenomenological/representative pole. "Humor" would then be conceived of as designating the psychic pole and the "comical," its expressive component, the representative pole.

This communication is established between one or some transmitters (the one, or ones, making others laugh) producing and transmitting the laughter-provoking message to one or some receivers (an individual or individuals or a group) who will respond by laughing (encoded facial-vocal communication), which itself acts as a laughter-provoking stimulus within a collectivity and

---

[1] Claude E. Shannon and Warren Weaver, *The Mathematical Theory of Communication*, Champaign IL: University of Illinois Press, 1998, p. 7.

conveys positive or negative feedback to the transmitter or transmitters. Let us point out that the transmitter and the receiver can be the same person.

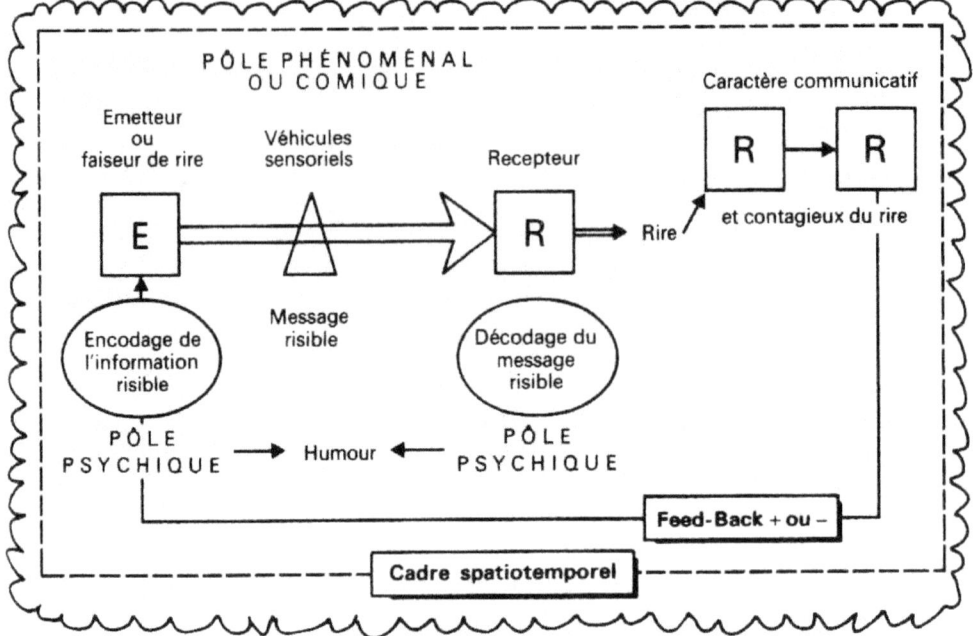

Winnicott's Third Area or Area of Illusion in which this laughable-laughter communication is plunged.

Translation of terms: Phenomenal or comical pole; Transmitter or the laughter-maker; Sensorial vehicle; Receiver; Laughter; Communicative, contagious nature of laughter; Encoding of laughter-provoking information; Laughter-provoking message; Decoding of the laughter-provoking message; Psychic pole; Humor; Psychic pole; Feedback + or -; Spatiotemporal setting

The laughable message is conveyed through different communication channels using different sensory modalities (sight, hearing, but also touch, or even, rarely, smell and taste).

To begin with let us state the categories of "sensory vehicles" of the laughter-provoking message.

3. **The categories of sensory vehicles of the laughter-provoking message.** I shall distinguish between verbal, non verbal and mixed (verbal and non-verbal) categories.

A) *The verbal categories* may be visual, therefore written, or acoustic, therefore oral. They are grouped together in what one might call the verbal comical. Included here are puns, anagrams, charades, palindromes, spoonerisms, witticisms. When these are based on thoughts, when they use words as vehicles of expression, one would then speak of wit and no longer of the verbal comical.

B) *The non-verbal categories* are or visual, acoustical or motor tactile.

a) The visual categories produce mime, pantomime, through mimetic-gesturing, caricature and humorous drawings using written forms, as well as through the pictorially or sculpturally laughable (comical objects, for example).

b) The acoustical categories open the way to musical jokes (see Mozart, Eric Satie, for example.) One may cite the unexpected, incongruous occurrence of "organic" noise such as growling stomachs, hiccups, flatulence, belches, but also voices whose tone or intensity is discordant in relation to the content of the discourse, as well as ventriloquists' performances.

c) The motor-tactile categories include tickling, other tactile, motor playing.

C) *The mixed categories* include both the verbal and non-verbal and can be particularly used in connection with comical situations and comical characters.

4. **The spatiotemporal setting.** –Laughter-provoking communication always takes place within a spatiotemporal, socio-cultural setting that may be specialized, institutionalized, becoming a laughter "sanctuary," or non-institutionalized.

A) *Laughter "sanctuaries."* –This institutionalization allows the free spreading of laughter and the laughable, which are authorized, even prescribed. One may cite:

a) Celebrations.- "Playful high points" of social life. In earlier times, there were the annual celebrations of "primitive" agrarian societies celebrating above all the end of winter and the return of spring with great playful ceremonies (the wearing of ceremonial costumes, dances, songs dedicated to fertility, games, pranks ending in orgies).

There also existed some celebrations institutionalized by those in power that strengthened the norms and laws by practicing "anti-acts," rituals involving a reversal of norms or dramatizing rebelliousness. The societies of Antiquity revealed a very ancient use of these mechanisms.

The annual Babylonian festival of the Sacaea featured a mock king with a dramatization of reversals of rank. Upon that occasion, a slave was hanged or crucified who had played the role of the sovereign, issuing orders, using the king's concubines, engaging in orgy or lust.

Georges Balandier has explained that this unleashed power was false power. It was shown theatrically in the form of a trouble-maker imposing the need to restore the reign of order, and it is in the name of this that the sacrifice of the false king is offered.[1]

- The Greek Kronia (annual festival).

- The Bacchanalia (celebrated in honor of Bacchus and solely consisting in pranks and libations) and the Roman Saturnalia.

In the Middle Ages, let us above all mention the Feast of Fools that took place between Christmas and the Feast of Kings, being held in cathedral towns and giving rise to the election of a bishop, pope or king of fools. This was a complete reversal of the usual way of being. The cathedral was then given over to the playful aggressiveness of the popular celebration. In addition, let us cite the carnival, another quite ritualized means of expression and popular liberation, fun fairs and other celebrations of all kinds.

b) Games. –They constitute the second major institutionalized setting. Whether a matter of ilinx (tobogganing, swinging), whirling (merry-go-rounds, racing), fiction (imitations-disguises), competitions-fights (sports), games of chance or sexual games, games can also find their place within a festive setting (the tickling contest during the festival of honey among the Guayaki Indians, for example). Laughter bursting out and spreading during the games can express a kind of joy linked to accomplishing individual motor feats, to victory in a competition (individual or collective), therefore to superiority over one's adversary, but also the pleasure of certain ways of poking fun exchanged in the course of playful interaction.

c) Rituals, the third setting. Certain rites can be the object of parody (cf. the sacred clowns of the Pueblo Indians (Hopi, Zuni)).

Otherwise, rites of passage (ceremonies celebrating the passage from one "existential state to another" such as birth, puberty, marriage, death) can be the

---

[1] Georges Balandier, *Le pouvoir sur scènes*, Paris: Balland, 1980.

occasion of festivities marked by the set of characteristics mentioned above, among them games, pranks, jokes, therefore of the laughable and of laughter (during meals, among other times). In *Sun Chief,* Don Talayesva gives two exemplary circumstances, upon the occasion of the *wowochim* or tribal initiation, and that of marriage (see above).

Therapeutic rituals, during which laughter is one of the instruments of therapy may also be cited.

d) Comic theater (direct laughter-provoking communication) has since ancient times constituted a temple of the laughable and of laughter with the comedies of Aristophanes, Plautus, Terence. At a much later period, we may cite the *commedia dell'arte*, Goldoni, the comedies of Molière, then the more recent works of Labiche, Feydeau, Courteline.

e) In very different cultural settings, let us remember the dances of the comical Katcinas and the Hopi sacred clowns.

f) Let us not forget the circus with its clowns, music hall shows, place of expression of cabaret singers, tellers of funny stories, stand-up comics, impersonators, mimes, ventriloquists.

g) Cinema, television are recent settings of indirect laughter-provoking communication with Charlie Chaplin, Buster Keaton, Laurel and Hardy, the Marx Brothers, Tati, just to cite a few great classic figures.

h) Finally, let us mention literature, whether it be oral, in traditional societies (the telling of myths, tales), or written (other indirect laughter-provoking communication through cartoons, satirical newspapers, novels).

Concerning comical myths, the collective imagination of the populations of North America invented a rather well-known character, the Trickster, who embodies a form of comical, social and political criticism. The African traditions also make room for a turbulent, laughable entity in their myths and tales. Indeed, certain myths have had Legba, a divine trickster, emerge as an intermediary between the gods and humanity. God of communication, with the gift of omnipresence, he sets his divine lack of discipline up against the discipline of the universal social order. He uses ruse, plays pranks, stirs up confusion. He is a wily god who makes people laugh.

B) *Non-institutionalized settings.*-Other, non-institutionalized, social settings within which pranks, jokes, jesting, laughter go on may authorize this form of communication. Social, friendly, family gatherings may incorporate some festive elements, over a meal, for example.

Everyday social activities (work or leisure) put people into contact belonging to the same or different (people/pets, men/women, adults/children, powerful people/subordinates) ontological categories. Jokes and situations of incompetence or inadequacy are then eminently laughter-provoking.

Joking relationships suggest certain types of family interaction propitious to laughter. In contrast to the respect and distance maintained between persons belonging to different categories (see the passage on the laughter of children in Africa), familiarity, joking, even insults are obligatory among certain members of a kinship group (clan, lineage, bloodline).

C) *Forbidden contexts*. —Certain culturally determined contexts may prohibit laughter: cemeteries, temples, for example.

5. **The transmitter or transmitters**. —They may be voluntary or involuntary.

A) *Involuntary "laughter-makers" are so without knowing it.* They may be human beings or animals "humanized" through a process of identification. Their mimetic gesturing, their behavior, talk, personality traits, conduct in certain specific situations may be laughable owing to their involuntary incongruousness and/or incompetence, their failure of bodily, verbal, behavioral, intellectual or emotional control.

B) *Those voluntarily producing the laughable.*

These are either amateurs (jokers, pranksters, teasers, funny personalities, witty people) gifted when it comes to playfulness, humorous creativity, exercising their talents in the domain of everyday life.

There are also the professionals. In this case, we call them comedians, living institutions of what is "aesthetically laughable," differing from the rudimentarily laughable through its sophisticated preparation, and especially through the techniques for producing it.

A certain number of those humorous comedians, no matter what their cultural milieu and the times in which they worked should be mentioned here. We shall see that they have enjoyed a quite specific social position and function.

a) The Jesters.

Ceremonial jesters (sacred). They are present in a great many societies established in North and Central America. Irony, parody, transgression define their unique position and their use. They introduce pranks into the sacred, playing in spectacles in which the most exacting ritual may coexist alongside mockery.

Domestic jesters, already found in Persia, Egypt, Greece, Rome, they were employed in the homes of rich and powerful people to make people laugh during meals, then, in the Middle Ages by barons and in the Church by abbots and bishops.

Court fools or jesters. They appear later on in the retinue of princes and kings where, by virtue of holding a position within the heart of the political institution, they are different in nature. It would not be until the XIVth century that the job of fool would become a special position. As Georges Balandier has explained, the fool and the prince served to show power from the dual perspective of force and derision, of fortune and misfortune; they form a dramatic pair. The fool has the privilege of saying everything and doing everything in terms of facetiousness and playing pranks.

The public jesters present a different picture, though the respective functions may overlap. They would also become "actors."

b) The circus ring, stage, television, movie screen present characters that overturn society's whole way of thinking, counter conventions and ordinary morality, use exaggeration and farce to uncover what is hidden.

They are clowns (characters of English farces, then circus clowns) burlesque comedians (of the theater/cinema, successors of the public jesters), music hall artists, but also tellers of funny tales.

c) Let us not forget the caricaturists, cartoonists, writers and satirists.

6. **The receiver or receivers, that is to say, the laughers.** Like any emotional facial mimicry, their laughter obeys rules of expression encoded by and for the group. Thus laughter is prescribed, authorized or prohibited depending on the subjects (according to age, gender, social status), the socio-cultural setting, the object of the laughable message, the intentions and the transmitter or transmitters (depending on age, gender, social status).

Undergirded by a system of representations and values, the social control exercised over engaging in laughter has also made it "conventional" and freed it from the affect of pleasure to take on new functions and meanings. In particular, we may cite polite laughter, embarrassed laughter, seductive laughter. Its technique is dependent both on cultural rules defined by each social group and on phenotypic, facial and vocal characteristics. This technique is in the service of expressing joy and basic pleasures, but also develops a whole set of "laughing" facial expressions having multiple valid functions and meanings within a given cultural context that are adopted by the members of the society in question. It thus plays a role in the cultural encoding of universal laughter, therefore generating "socialized" forms of laughter.

The social functions must be elucidated by taking into account other elements of the system of which it is a part. Nevertheless, allow me to state some of them:

- expression of individual joy and psychic security engendered by the group's social cohesion;

- symbolic sanctioning of deviancy and eccentricity, constituting a very effective means of social control of mores;

- means of avoiding negative sanctioning, punishment by inhibiting the aggressiveness of other persons;

- instrument of politeness;

- instrument of defense against anxiety;

- instrument of social exclusion;

- instrument of seduction and affective pursuits.

7. **Themes and techniques of laughter.**

A) It seems that the comical production undergirded by a complex system of representations, beliefs and values, is also encoded, subject therefore to prescribed rules and prohibitions. This code is quite clearly common to the transmitter and the receiver(s). The prohibitions may concern deaths, ancestors, illnesses, misfortunes (bound to the cultural context), while what is prescribed is aimed at the one or ones foreign to the group, deviants, language. Moreover, despite the variability of these objects, there is a high probability of identifying invariant factors in the object of the laughter-provoking message.

Indeed, it always seems to reach human beings in their activities, accomplishments, character; society as regards its order, its hierarchy, its institutions, its rules, its values, the logic of its functioning; non-humans, be they "humanized" animals or objects. Certain laughter-provoking objects constitute invariants:

-   the one or ones foreign to the group of laughers;

-   deviants or eccentrics within a group;

-   political power, the social order and all established authority, all institutions;

-   sexuality;

-   language.

B) These objects become the playthings of playful and laughable transformations through the use of multiple techniques "borrowed" in particular from the rhetorical figures of speech, of which may be named: hyperbole (exaggeration), litotes (understatement), metaphor, metonymy, repetition, inversion, irony.

Also used are certain effects of contrast such as burlesquing, parodying, sexual language (highly degrading). This play of transformations of the object or practice of mockery leads both to cognitive effects such as surprise, nonsense, incongruity, but also to distinct debasement or symbolic aggression of it, as well as to its inability to adapt to society. Thus, human beings may be "mechanized," treated as things, animalized, animals or objects may be "humanized," adults infantilized, children metamorphosed into adults, men depicted as women, or women as men in a reversal of roles. Change of ontological or social category is a very effective way of generating the laughable, therefore laughter.

8. **Functions of this laughter-provoking communication.** All the writers on the subject attribute five functions to this type of social communication to which a type of humor is associated. Three psychic functions can in fact be identified:

-   the first would aim at the symbolic satisfaction of sadistic drives by clearly degrading the object, this being accompanied by the expression of narcissistic triumph (aggressive humor);

-   the second would aim at the symbolic satisfaction of exhibitionistic and/or voyeuristic drives through verbal language and/or the visual representation of obscene humor.

- the third would be defensive with regard to anxiety-provoking existential facts and topics (black humor and self-mockery);

- to these I would add an intellectual function generating pleasure through the transgression of the rules of rational logic, through wordplay and the absurd;

- finally, I shall mention all the social functions:

  * exclusion of the person or persons foreign to the group, with the concomitant strengthening of "social narcissism;"

  * exclusion of what is deviant with the maintaining and strengthening of rules and conventions protective of the social order;

  * social and political criticism;

  * acquisition of prestige.

For my part, I shall add as a complement the notion of the "psychic homeostasis of a society." Indeed, the laughable and laughter are tools at the service of the "psychic homeostasis" of a group. Any society in search of mental equilibrium by way of the (direct and symbolic) satisfaction of drives, objects of repression of greater or lesser significance, would have available for these ends, among other means, this fundamentally playful, transgressive institutionalized laughable/laughter system resorting to a language of childhood and procuring an economic gain in pleasure expressed in laughter.

Thus the laughable and laughter manifestly take on multiple forms, multiple functions, and multiple meanings. Their relationships to play and transgression are clear. One writer on the subject, Eric Blondel, considers that laughter and playing are related to one another through pleasure, suspending reality, transgressing norms and substituting new rules, freedom and childhood or the return to childhood. For him, laughter is born out of a hiatus, a break in serious, everyday social time.[1]

---

[1] Eric Blondel, *Le risible et le dérisoire*, Paris: Presses Universitaires de France, 1988.

CONCLUSION

Thus, after having envisioned the threefold encoding of laughter (biological, psychical and socio-cultural), a new picture has emerged. The distance that was initially taken with regard to the reductionist scientific, uninformed discourse on the subject has now found legitimate justification. Ideas about its being specific to human beings, about its being the facial expression of Joy indicative of good health, as well its spontaneous execution are henceforth outmoded.

Manufactured in a remarkably sophisticated fashion, laughter seems to be the product of a multidimensional (phylogenetic, ontogenetic, cultural and individual) history within which its relationship to playing proves to be structural in nature.

In virtue of its belonging to the system of laughable communication, at once playful in scope in structure, functions and meanings, laughter seems to preserve this archaic relation to playing in which it would represent its "mimetic partner." It would then be a matter of the mimicry of play specific to human beings, signaling the abandonment of serious, constraining reality for that third area, that of illusion and of "freedom." It would also express a composite kind of pleasure depending on the circumstances: that of mastery and narcissistic triumph rooted in painful experiences; that of the symbolic satisfaction of partial, sadistic and voyeuristic drives; that of super ego transgression and seduction. However, laughter also has its place within the system of emotional, individual and social forms of expression.

Within the first, it communicates affective messages inherent in the psychic experience of laughing subjects. Positive when their moods are playful, joyful, following some expected, or even unexpected, personal or collective success, laughter is a sign of narcissistic triumph and the pleasure of mastery.

Nevertheless, it can also be a defense mechanism against distressing and painful affects that it endeavors to reject or deny by representing the "mimetic opposite." It is in this way that it indirectly transmits negative affective messages.

Finally, channel of facial-respiratory discharge, it permits the remarkable outflow of a quantum of (psychically uncontrollable) psychic excitation or tension.

In the second, it is a matter of an "encoded" social laughter or "laughing mimicry" that is disconnected and freed from any personal affect, communicating from that point on "collective emotions" prescribed in certain specific types of social interaction and in this way participating in a group's repertory of conventional social mimicry. Hence these emotions obey the rules of politeness and good manners. For example, there is the laughter of "prescribed" collective joy and satisfaction, polite laughter, the laughter of seduction, or even of dissimulated embarrassment.

Out of universal laughter, the phylogenetic legacy of the mimicry of the social play of the higher primates, human beings would thus have created its polymorphism, its functional versatility and its diversity of meanings, therefore its variability through the elaboration of social rules, pure creations of human mental activity generating a new marker of social identity.

Finally, above and beyond its belonging to systems of laughable and emotional communication, it definitely seems that laughter also plays a role in the fundamental drama of human existence constituted by the processes of life/deadly processes antagonism.

Indeed, as a defense against death and its deadly processes, the facial-vocal metaphor that laughter embodies would perhaps be that of a triumphant outburst of life.

Thus a burst of laughter would represent a fleeting burst of life....

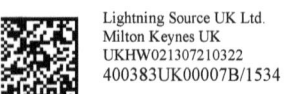

9 781848 901193